Killing

Her

Cancer

By: S. Heinson

Book Cover by <a href="https://www.vecteezy.com/free-photos/ai-generated">Ai Generated Stock photos by Vecteezy</a>

Translated using Microsoft Word.

First edition May 2024

For Chelsi

I'm glad you decided to stick around.

I would like to take a moment to thank Patricia Hernandez for proof reading the Spanish version. For giving your approval, and for sending food for me all the time. Thank you very much, from the bottom of my stomach, to the top of my heart.

:S.

Menu

Appetizer

Hello,

I'd like to tell you about the time my wife had ovarian cancer. A 22-mm malignant tumor, to be precise. I'd also like to tell you how we killed it. At home. Without the use of "drugs". Using only what Mother Nature has provided us with. In an easily digestible way. To the best of my knowledge, with every backing document I can provide. From the many late- night hours of my research. These are my notes:

* THIS IS NOT MEDICAL ADVICE *

This is merely my experience and I hope this finds you well. Now, let's start with a little background information and an introduction. All of the resources contained in this book are linked. The rest is my opinion. This is not medical advice. I am only here to offer a bit of perspective on an approach to healing. It is truly only my opinion that there are plenty of amazing doctors. There are also many that have no intent on actually healing. They laugh off some of the older practices which would actually bring them around to the root cause of a lot of our health issues. Like taking stool samples from every cancer

patient and checking for parasites to rule them out. It is a pretty simple test and those little bastards can cause a lot of our health issues.
CDC: 60+ Million Americans Are Infected With Sneaky Parasites — How One Woman Cured Them Naturally

Yahoo is part of the Yahoo family of brands. (n.d.). https://www.yahoo.com/lifestyle/cdc-60-million-americans-infected

Then, they come with the bandages, drugs, and all of these "solutions" they have to offer, which typically involve killing you a little bit, in a different way, on an "individual, case-by-case basis," of course.

I enjoy watching the commercials for the new drugs and waiting for the side effects. They always show some happy-go-lucky people living their happy-go-lucky lives, while they describe these horrible, random side-effects that have nothing to do with what they are applying this new patch to. (I think it's messed up when the side-effect of their medicine happens to be the same damn thing you were taking it for.) And what it "may cause." They always start out with some random problem that I wasn't aware we needed prescriptions for. "Do you have a problem with urinating in public?" Then, they pitch their drug. And here comes the run-down. "Users might experience headaches, dizziness, drowsiness,

diarrhea, and so on and so-forth. Then comes the good stuff. "Hair loss, leprosy, kidney failure, blood in urine, bloody stools, tooth and bone decay, random thoughts of suicide, night terrors..."
Why do we want to take the pills they push? Do we ever stop and ask these people, "What are you trying to do to me?" No. We typically trust our doctors. If we ask for clarification, it may leave us more confused than before we asked the question. And they make sure to use their technological terms, which most people don't have a ready-to-fire definition of. Most people don't ask for a definition of the words that they don't understand either. We tend to use "word implication or association" opposed to word definitions. Thanks to our public education system. Or, we're too busy trying to comprehend the news we just received. Not all doctors overload people with information and crazy words right away, but a lot do. It is sabotage. It is also old and tiring to keep up with.
Let me sum it up in the best way, that I myself, have had it summed up for as well. As a medical doctor, all they are allowed to do is three things:

- **Prescribe medications**
- **Perform surgeries**
- **Offer Advice.**   That is all ladies and gentleman.

Did you ever notice that a medical doctor typically will not suggest a chiropractor? And vice versa. And then, neither of them will typically recommend a therapist. It is pretty funny though. After we killed her cancer with her diet, I had asked a doctor about how important our diet was. He shook it off and said "Eh, as long as you're getting most of what you need, you're going to be fine." Then, when I asked about using our diet to heal? He responded with the usual "There isn't enough evidence to support any claims." Weird. I found a bunch of evidence. Endless pages of evidence. Claims from people that have successfully healed themselves and apparently, their information and data do not matter? Sounds about right. Since no one believes "people", I went to the science for my sources. I thought "doctors" did too. Apparently not. Most people seem to get slapped around by everyone when they get diagnosed with cancer. It typically starts in the damn doctors' office. Although, the topic of this book is no laughing matter, if you lack a sense of humor, I strongly suggest finding one as we move forward. Because laughing is my defense mechanism. The absurdity of that which I have come to realize, through my experience with the revelations I incurred, during this time period was certainly too much to handle at times, and I had to begin to laugh again.

I have provided as much information in the most condensed version as possible, with links for you to follow. Please do your own research. The more you know your body, the easier it is to heal it. And you are the only one who can save yourself. We all want easy answers for all of our questions. Well, here it is. And it couldn't be easier. What we eat either helps us or hurts us. There is no in-between. I will say it again. What we eat either hurts us or helps us. It is, in fact, black and white. There is no gray area whatsoever. We have many food scanner apps that we can use to check our foods today. They give you information on the harmful chemicals that are in all of your foods, makeup, etc. Most of us unknowingly ingest harmful, dangerous chemicals daily. We just don't know that we do. The buyer-beware laws in the U.S. are there to protect corporations. Not us. It's not "their" fault we didn't know the chemicals in our foods have horrible long-term side effects. And it's certainly not their fault we didn't know where a lot of the ingredients for the mass produced "vitamins" come from. Let me tell you, my friends.

YOU WILL BE SURPRISED.

The facts are that the citric acid found in most supplements is actually derived from mold. I found that top brand cereals contain what is called Trisodium phosphate or (TSP). Did you know that it's a commercial degreaser and you can purchase it at your local hardware store to clean your floors and drains? Your B12 vitamin supplements are sometimes derived from sewer water sludge. Now technically our bodies make B12 in our own kind of personal sewer sludge from our bellies. It actually, I believe ends up on our teeth in the mornings. Which is why, if you take a big drink of water when you wake up, you will get a little energy burst. It is from the B12 that just built up on your teeth overnight. Would you like to know where the vitamin D3 supplements come from? We take this one when we're too lazy to go outside and get some sun. Lanolin is a waxy substance that is secreted from the glands of sheep. It helps protect the sheep's skin, and it is used for our vitamin D3 supplement. Gelatin is a tasteless, pale powder that is derived from animal collagen, the protein of animal connective tissues. It is typically derived from the hides and bones of cattle as well as pigskin. Gummies of every kind use this.

You will be interested to know where your vanilla flavoring comes from.

Top 5 Weirdest Supplement Ingredients. (n.d.). Holtraceuticals. https://holtraceuticals.com/blogs/news/top-5-weirdest-supplement-ingredients

Vanilla "natural" flavoring is definitely natural. So is your raspberry flavoring, as well as a few others. Yet they are from the same animal. It is typically not derived from a plant. It is called castoreum, and it is used in food items, drinks and a favorite in liquors. Remember all of those yummy vanilla frappé drinks?

Castoreum: Also known as beaver anal gland juice. This additive is excreted from the caster sacs of mature North American and European beavers. This ingredient can be found on food listed as "natural flavoring." Castoreum can be found in foods that need vanilla, raspberry, or strawberry flavoring such as ice cream, yogurt, and instant oatmeal.

L-cysteine: L-cystine is a non-essential amino acid made from dissolved human hair or duck feathers. It is often used in commercial dough conditioners.

Carmine: Simply put, crushed bugs. This bright red food color is made from the crushed abdomen of female African beetles. This ingredient may also be listed at Natural Red #4. It can be found in red candies like Skittles, red tinted yogurts and juices like ones listed as ruby red.

S. (2013, September 11). 8 Food Additives That May Gross You Out. The Organic Dietitian. https://theorganicdietitian.com/8-food-additives-that-may-gross-you-out/

You read that right. There's more. And a lot of it. We wonder why we're constantly having strange

ailments. I have many more examples of why we need to eat the actual, naturally occurring foods our world has provided us with, since the beginning of time. We do not need all of the drugs and supplements they shove down our throats. And I don't want to eat or drink beaver anal gland juice anymore. That's just a messed-up string of words to have to say. Stranger Danger! I need an adult. This is not okay ladies and gentlemen.

Now. Let's talk cancer. Let's talk about how it *dies.* Unless... letting some guy, who's practicing at his job, pump you full of drugs that'll kill your entire immune system so they can stick you full of another radioactive chemical that kills your bodies ecosystem, maybe even you as well, sounds like a good idea. Then you need to stop reading this and grab a good self-help book. You deserve better. Back to cancer cell death. It cannot survive in an alkaline environment. Cancer cannot survive in an oxygenated or hydrogenated environment. These are facts proven through case studies noted in "The Sauce." Some of you may recall this information from science class. What is an alkaline environment? It is an environment that stays above 6.0 on the pH. scale. What does that mean? Our bodies are like an aquarium. If you have ever had a

pet fish, you may understand a little about water pH. (I used to have fish and knew these terms, but I didn't really comprehend what "ph." actually stood for.)

If you've walked into a convenience store, you've probably seen the water bottles that say ph. 9+. The "ph." on the water bottles stands for potential hydrogen. Hydrogen. Sound familiar? An item the military uses for bombs, perhaps? There have been studies showing that hydrogenated water can reduce tumors and cancers.

As medical science continues to advance, molecular hydrogen has started to find its way into oncology. Colorectal cancer is a common cause of death due to cancer, and removal of tumors is still the mainstay of treatment. Hydrogen-rich water did show anti-cancer properties in a study. With its antioxidant properties and ability to decrease oxidative stress, it could be a potential game changer in the future. A combination of hydrogen-rich water and 5-fluorouracil (5-FU) did show improvement in the size of the tumor, fibrosis, and content of collagen. Another systematic review was to see molecular hydrogen's effect as an adjunctive therapy for cancer treatment. A total of 677 articles were reviewed, and were selected for final review. Hydrogen was noted to have potential in treatment, overall prognosis, quality of life, and tumor reduction. Hydrogen-rich water's effect on exercise capacity and physical endurance is of particular interest to individuals with a fondness for physical activity. Additionally, the potential for a positive impact on cardiovascular function can reduce the risk of heart disease. Additionally, the possible effect of hydrogen-rich water on mental health is intriguing, with the initial results being encouraging. Also, its effect on anti-cancer properties holds promise in the field of oncology. Given its potential to positively impact liver function, anti-aging, and oxidative stress, hydrogen-rich water is a subject of ongoing research and growing interest. Hydrogen-rich water offers several potential strengths, including its antioxidant, anti-inflammatory, and anti-apoptotic properties. It can also help decrease oxidative stress. Some studies showed that it may also improve physical endurance, cognitive function, and overall well-being.

National Center for Biotechnology Information (NCBI)[Internet]. Bethesda (MD): National Library of Medicine (US), National Center for Biotechnology Information; [1988] – [cited 2024 May 18]. Available from: https://www.ncbi.nlm.nih.gov/pmc/articles/PMC10816294/#:~:text=As%20medical%20science,reduction%20%5B28%5D

With these findings I have come to believe that we may be some sort of electric battery that runs off of oxygenated hydrogen. Possibly.

If you have ever owned a freshwater aquarium, then you should know that your water pH should be neutral at 6.0; if it's too low or high, your fish will die. The water has now become toxic. If the water tests lower than 6.0 pH, it most likely has a lot of fish waste built up. Maybe the filter needs to be changed. If your water isn't cleaned of the chemicals from your tap water, it will kill the fish. If it develops bacteria in the tank, it will kill the fish. If you fill your aquarium full of soda and alcohol, it will kill the fish. It has the same effect on us. If you have never owned an aquarium, then now you know. Don't feed the fish beer and soda. Do you see where I am going, ladies and gentlemen? This is just for our energy. We should all understand that our bodies water pH is not the same as our blood PH. We will go further. Although there are many possible ways to fight cancer, it starts with the pH of our blood, which is affected by the digestion process of the liquids we drink and also, the foods that we eat. In "The Sauce," links are provided for foods that cause our bodies blood pH to alter. We all have our own little environment inside of us. Our own personal terrarium. It's up to us if we make it functional and beneficial. At the same time. It is up to us if we decide to neglect it and let it rot.

Throughout the last 5 years or so, my wife had a hard time getting her cancer diagnosed. She went to the doctor to address her health concerns, as most responsible adults would. Stomach pains, abnormal periods, and more would be reported to the "doctors." But they told her it was irritable bowel syndrome. They told her it was Crohn's disease, stress, and her diet (which was true), but it took her getting pregnant and not stopping bleeding every month before we were able to find out what was going on inside of her body. She was pregnant with twins. We were ecstatic. We were trying actively. Unfortunately, we lost them after 4 months into the pregnancy. We were sad, yes. I was more than happy to be able to create some babies with her. Before we lost them and during the pregnancy, she continued getting her period. We were sent in for a transvaginal ultrasound, and that was when the tumor was detected in her ovaries and it was malignant. Unfortunately, due to the medical system protocols, they did the scope and took their data and information and refused to tell my wife what was happening in there. It's so impersonal how they treat us and the way they work. The nurse saw the mass. She gasped. My wife got excited. She thought it was still about the babies. She really thought they were making sure the babies were okay because she is small in stature and had so many issues.

Twins are an understandably scary thought for her. So, she left. Still thinking she was okay. After a few days and no information, she turned to me and said, "Maybe I need to up my life insurance. What if I die giving birth to your big-ass babies?" I agreed. She made the appointment with her life insurance company. We went. And it was during that meeting that my wife was informed that she had cancer. Not from her doctor. Not in some heartfelt setting like you see in the movies. Her insurance agent was the one who told her as she was being denied the additional coverage. Now I will make mention, that her insurance company actually did eventually approve her requested coverage, as she had technically not been diagnosed by a doctor that she had cancer yet. It was all around a horrible experience. After years of misdiagnosis leading to what ended up being cancer, you have to find out from your life insurance agent while you are being denied coverage while also basically finding out your babies are dying at the same time. This place sucks. I hate our system. Upon finally getting in to the doctor, during the diagnosis, we found that the twins were lost and a tumor was in her ovaries. It was 22mm and second stage. That was heartbreaking. But in the end, I know if she hadn't gotten pregnant, they most likely wouldn't have caught it, and I would not be telling you *this* version of the story.

Now, the tumor. 22mm is almost an inch around. Which is about the size of a bottle cap or a U.S. quarter dollar. A quick note for encouragement. After 5 months, it was documented at 0mm. All they had offered her was chemotherapy. She declined it. She was already aware of some of the side effects of chemotherapy. After finding out she had cancer, we became aware of all of the side effects. If you haven't really taken a dive into the course of chemo, let me enlighten you. First, they take you off all vitamins. Because you cannot have a functioning immune system for their drugs to work.

What happens when you kill your immune system? You now have no defense against the bacteria and viruses that we constantly come into contact with. For the ones that refuse to wash their hands after using a restroom, to the ones that take no consideration of the effect of their personal hygiene:

Cellulitis a common, potentially serious bacterial skin infection. Bacteria, Viruses, and Parasites are the primary inhabitants related to poor hygiene and they are the ones that cause deadly infectious diseases. These deadly germs use the human body as a host for reproduction and multiplying in no time thereby forcing the body succumb to their act.

Diarrhea: The simple act of washing hands with soap and water can cut diarrheal disease by one-third.

Cholera is an acute bacterial infection of the intestinal tract. It causes severe attacks of diarrhea that, without treatment, can quickly lead to acute dehydration and death. Cholera can be prevented by access to sanitation, safe drinking water, and good hygiene behavior.

Trachoma is an eye infection which starts as pink eye and is spread mainly through poor hygiene caused by lack of adequate water and unsafe environmental sanitation conditions, such as inability to wash hands. About 6 million people are blind today because of trachoma. It affects women two to three times more than men. Children are also especially susceptible.

Freebeck, M. (2022, June 2). Hygiene Implications on Health — Simply the Basics: The Nation's Premier Hygiene Bank. Simply the Basics: The Nation's Premier Hygiene Bank. https://www.simplythebasics.org/blog/hygieneimplicationsonhealth

If you are undergoing chemotherapy, these are some of the challenges you will face if you only USE THE RESTROOM. It doesn't stop there. That's just the initial step into the world after you leave the session. You still have to suffer some or all of the side effects of chemotherapy itself. Which of the lists is interesting to decipher? Most of us look at the first option that our search engine pulls up, which doesn't seem terrible from a possible outsider's perspective. "You get super skinny and lose your hair, but not your life." Unfortunately, that is not always the case, and it doesn't stop there. That's just where our blinders get put up, as if there are no other options. Let's discuss the warnings about handling the drugs alone.

Chemotherapy drugs are considered to be hazardous to people who handle them or come into contact with them. For patients, this means the drugs are strong enough to damage or kill cancer cells. But this also means the drugs can be a concern for others who might be exposed to them. You may notice special clothing and protective equipment being worn by the nurses and other members of your cancer care team. Pharmacists and nurses who prepare chemo drugs use a special type of pharmacy that must meet certain regulations. And nurses and others who give your chemo and help take care of you afterwards wear protective clothing, such as 2 pairs of special gloves and a gown, and sometimes goggles or a face shield. If you're getting IV chemo, there might be a disposable pad under the infusion tubing to protect the surface of the bed or chair.

Chemotherapy Safety. (n.d.). American Cancer Society.
https://www.cancer.org/cancer/managing-cancer/treatment-types/chemotherapy/chemotherapy-safety.html#

They want you to let them put a chemical in you that you're not supposed to touch. People have to wear special protective gear to administer it to you. Now, you have to isolate yourself from your friends and family so they don't get sick from being in contact with your body fluids if you share a restroom. So, if you don't have a home with two bathrooms, you are now in the middle of another problem. You have now been isolated, with no support system left at that point. After dealing with all of this, you now have the long-term effects. Fatigue, heart problems, infertility, hair loss, neuropathy, lung problems and more. The one side effect of chemo they tend to save for last though is CANCER. A side effect of your cancer treatment is CANCER. Something's wrong here.

I'd like to take the time to note that getting healthier by eating proper foods does not have these results and effects. I feel like I just needed to point that out. We need to understand what our "hot chips" and flavored drinks really do to our bodies. We'll dig into the health issues they cause further in the book.

Once she declined the chemotherapy, they were seemingly uninterested in her return to health after that. Until the end, when they suggested a holistic doctor. After the fact that we had already put it into remission at home with the holistic information I was learning. It's like, if you don't let them kill you themselves, they get sad about it. No contact. No phone calls were returned. We were on our own. Even some parts of her family got weird. The real ones stayed true as they always do. But most of them still wanted her to go party and drink, you know... pretend like everything is fine, so *they* weren't uncomfortable about her dying. Or maybe it was to finish the job. That is still unclear. When she declined. No bs. They got salty. No one came by to check on her. Just to check on her, without their own guilt playing their hand. What a shame. Most of her "friends" disappeared. Only a few, true friends made her answer the phone and get out of bed. They know who they are. Their deeds do not go unappreciated from a caring husbands' perspective. That is not uncommon, apparently, from what I've gathered from others. Want to know if you have true friends? Get cancer. Want to know what kind of family you actually surround yourself with? Get cancer. And with the doctors, it's the same. If you don't jump on board, you're on your own. Doctors don't want to be questioned. Just shut up and do as you're told. Just a question to think about and ask yourself. Why do they call what a "doctor" does a practice? Is it because they just couldn't get it perfect? And why do they keep telling us what we need to be by calling us patients? Is it like a subliminal, mk-ultra, television-type suggestive projection into our subconscious? I'm still working that one out. I guess I need to keep practicing and be more patient...

During this time period, I was still the owner and only employee of my company. All day long, 10 to 12 hours a day, I was trading my labor for debt. At night. I started reading. EVERYTHING. I had to know. I couldn't rest knowing my wife was dying, lying next to me. It wasn't fair. How am I supposed to sleep at a time like that? What kind of "man" could I call myself, just going to sleep while my wife lay there dying? I couldn't. I tried. I could not allow myself to sleep or eat, really. I had no idea what to do. So, I read. Everything. I just knew I wouldn't rest until I had her healthy again. If she was dying, then I would die trying. I'd sleep for maybe two or three hours, and then my eyes were back open. Typically, it was 4:30. Every morning. I woke up. No matter how little sleep I got. It did not matter. After reading every possible article and book that I could find on self-healing. I still wasn't satisfied. One day. I was working. It was another annoying Monday, I believe. I looked around at the job I've done for two decades and knew. I could happily walk away from it if given the opportunity. I enjoy what I do. I enjoy helping people out and not screwing them over. I once slept well at night. And on that night, I made my decision.

I went signed up for school. Holistic healing and natural medicine. I kept finding all of these options that help us live longer and more naturally without all the "foods" we've been duped into eating for almost every meal of the day. I had to pursue this knowledge. Unfortunately, but fortunately, school started with psychophysiology. The timing was perfect as I needed the mental help as well. I was now left learning more but still having to pursue killing her cancer.

Throughout our journey, we found that it requires being very honest with "who" you are, how long you would like to live, and how well you'd like to do it. The more I studied and learned, the more I wasn't getting satisfaction. I learned that almost all of our skin care and beauty products are killing us as well. They have us rubbing all of their chemicals on our skin, and as it absorbs and distributes inside of us, it can give us cancer as well.

Look at your ingredients on the bottles if you don't believe me. See for yourself that they most likely contain propylene glycol variants like PEG-10:

Accumulating evidence suggests that PEG10 plays an important role in tumor growth in various cancers, including hepatocellular carcinoma, lung cancer and prostate cancer.

Li, X., Xiao, R., Tembo, K., Hao, L., Xiong, M., Pan, S., Yang, X., Yuan, W., Xiong, J., & Zhang, Q. (2016, February 23). PEG10 promotes human breast cancer cell proliferation, migration and invasion. International Journal of Oncology. https://www.spandidos-publications.com/10.3892/ijo.2016.3406

It's not just in shampoo. I found it in:

- anti-aging
- around-eye cream
- BB cream
- beach & sport sunscreen
- blush
- bronzer/highlighter
- brow liner
- CC cream

- concealer
- conditioner
- eye liner
- eye shadow
- facial moisturizer/treatment
- foundation
- hair spray
- hair styling aide
- hair treatment/serum
- lip balm
- lip gloss
- lip liner
- lipstick
- makeup primer
- mascara
- mask
- moisturizer
- moisturizer with SPF
- serums & essences
- setting powder/spray
- styling mousse/foam and more.

Although they say propylene glycol non variants are safe. I think it deserves some attention since there is evidence that suggests otherwise: The toxicity in children. Although PG is generally considered safe, when used in high doses or for prolonged periods,

PG toxicity can occur. Reported adverse effects from PG include central nervous system (CNS) toxicity, hyperosmolarity, hemolysis, cardiac arrhythmia, seizures, agitation, and lactic acidosis. Patients at risk for toxicity include infants, those with renal or hepatic insufficiency, epilepsy, and burn patients receiving extensive dermal applications of PG containing products. Laboratory monitoring of PG levels, osmolarity, lactate, pyruvate, bicarbonate, creatinine, and anion gap can assist practitioners in making the diagnosis of PG toxicity. Numerous studies and case reports have been published on PG toxicity in adults. National Center for Biotechnology Information (NCBI)[Internet]. Bethesda (MD): National Library of Medicine (US), National Center for Biotechnology Information; [1988] – [cited 2024 May 18]. Available from: https://www.ncbi.nlm.nih.gov/pmc/articles/PMC4341412/#

If you haven't read your shampoo bottle or soap bottles, you may want to start. Look up the side effects of all the ingredients like:

Sodium Lauryl Sulfate

Hair loss The CIR report1 is also cited as supporting the claim that SLS can cause hair loss and baldness.13,16,32 The CIR report states as follows:

Autoradiographic studies of rat skin treated with radiolabeled Sodium Lauryl Sulfate found heavy deposition of the detergent on the skin surface and in the hair follicles; damage to the hair follicle could result from such deposition.

National Center for Biotechnology Information (NCBI)[Internet]. Bethesda (MD): National Library of Medicine (US), National Center for Biotechnology Information; [1988] – [cited 2024 May 18]. Available from: https://www.ncbi.nlm.nih.gov/pmc/articles/PMC4651417/

No matter how much knowledge I attained, I still kept waking up. I could not sleep. I switched it up and then began to read the Bible when I woke up. I had officially run out of ideas. I'd say, "Alright. How do I do this? What am I missing? I know I do not know enough." I would open it to random pages and begin reading. I have already read it front to back in the past. Then, I opened the Bible one night, and to be honest, I have no idea which chapter I read. I read so many at that time. I know it brought me to Wormwood. That name spoke to me. I guess it was because it seems everything is going backwards. What "they" say is okay for us is bad. And then the Bible calls it out as bad. Naturally, I did a little digging, and that led me to find out how it is used to kill cancer cells. Only then did I feel like I had my answer. Does that mean everything is backwards and upside down? Possibly. Regardless of whether the world is backwards or not, the best guidance I think I received when it came to religion is this: If you have ever been praying and it just doesn't feel like your prayers are being heard, know that they are being heard. It's just that your plans and God's plans don't quite match up. We have to bend to God's plan. Because God is not going to bend for you. Change your path and intentions and see how life will change for you. I learned then what control I have and what I don't. I believe we are in control of ourselves. That's it. We don't understand the level of damage the foods we are putting into our bodies causes us. Because of the foods, drinks and everything we consume is so readily available. Everything we eat is premade. Down to baking a cake. A simple item to bake from scratch.

1 cup white sugar, ½ cup unsalted butter

2 large eggs, 2 teaspoons vanilla extract*****

1 ½ cups all-purpose flour, 1 ¾ teaspoons baking powder

½ cup milk

S. (2023, November 11). Simple White Cake. Allrecipes.
https://www.allrecipes.com/recipe/17481/simple-white-cake/

The suggested substitute for sugar is honey and the rule of thumb: For every 1 cup of sugar, substitute 1/2 to 2/3 cup honey. For every 1 cup of honey you use, subtract 1/4 cup of the other liquids from the recipe.

The beaver butt juice is your choice.

Let us take a look at what one of the top brand name box-cake ingredients has hidden in a cake for you.

Enriched Flour Bleached which is: wheat flour, niacin, iron, thiamin mononitrate, riboflavin, folic acid. And it has Sugar, Corn Syrup, Leavening, which is typically baking soda, sodium aluminum phosphate, monocalcium phosphate. Dicalcium Phosphate, Modified Corn Starch, Corn Starch, Propylene Glycol Mono and Diesters, Salt, Monoglycerides, Palm Oil, Sodium Stearoyl Lactylate, Xanthan Gum, Cellulose Gum, Natural and Artificial Flavor, and don't forget the Yellows 5 & 6.

Happy Birthday to you!

People ask for help, and it seems no one stops and thinks to themselves: "Maybe I need to start at home with myself and get better before I ask God or anyone else to stop everything they have going on and to come and help my ass get through life." Maybe stop and think about the fact that "all of these "foods" I keep shoving down my throat every day are poisoning me and making me a miserable, hormonal, out-of-shape wreck. They are literally killing me, slowly, as I fall apart." It is not God's fault. It's our fault. It was my own fault. I know this.

That's okay, too. They say, "Don't fix it if it isn't broke." Well, it was broken. I had to fix it. The first step would be knowledge. Actually, the first step is just the first step. No matter which direction taken. We can't ask for our problems to miraculously disappear. That is a nice fantasy. Unfortunately, that is all it will ever be. Learning a little bit goes a long way.

I also learned to listen a little better. It has been helpful to be quiet. Listening to the world and letting it guide me where I need to be. Not necessarily what I had in mind for my life's entire plan. I figure, why not?

During these times, my wife slept a lot. Although she was getting better. She was gaining her strength. We had no idea what was happening inside of her. I kept learning. Reading. Finding out that other people are suffering from the same treatment from the medical field. It has to stop. All it takes is for us to wake up and read our nutrition labels. Know the poisons we consume daily. Stop ingesting this garbage and start demanding change. Why do we take toothpaste advice from people who make their living off of our bad teeth?

According the American dental Association website:

All toothpastes with the ADA Seal of Acceptance must contain fluoride.

Toothpastes. (n.d.). American Dental Association. https://www.ada.org/en/resources/ada-library/oral-health-topics/toothpastes

The 13 best toothpastes for clean, healthy teeth in 2024

American Dental Association Seal of Acceptance: Oral care products like toothpaste, floss, mouthwash and manual and electric toothbrushes can earn the ADA's Seal of Acceptance. In order to do so, brands submit scientific evidence showing that their products meet specific safety and efficacy criteria, which the ADA evaluates. All ADA-approved toothpastes contain fluoride and are not made with flavoring agents that can cause or contribute to tooth decay, like sugar. This doesn't mean toothpastes without the ADA's Seal of Acceptance are ineffective — it just means brands have not voluntarily submitted their products for the ADA to review.

Fluoride: All of the experts we spoke to recommend choosing a toothpaste that contains fluoride, a cavity-fighting ingredient. Three types of fluoride may be listed on toothpaste ingredient labels, all of which are equally effective: sodium fluoride, stannous fluoride and sodium monofluorophosphate.

Sodium lauryl sulfate: Sodium lauryl sulfate, commonly referred to as SLS, is an ingredient found in many toothpastes that acts as a detergent for your teeth, says Dr. Lana Rozenberg, dentist and founder of Rozenberg Dental NYC. It's also what makes some toothpastes foamy. People can be sensitive to SLS, so if you are, look for an SLS-free toothpaste.

Texture: You'll commonly find toothpaste texture broken down into gels and pastes. Gel toothpastes have a smooth, non-foamy texture and are typically not abrasive or gritty. Paste toothpastes, on the

other hand, tend to be more foamy, thicker, grittier and solid in color, says Rozenberg.

Specialized options: Beyond protecting teeth from cavities, toothpaste can offer additional benefits like teeth whitening or enamel repair. Some are also designed for those with sensitive teeth. A toothpaste's packaging and label will say what it specifically targets, so think about whether that aligns with your teeth's needs.

Flavor: Toothpaste flavor is entirely a personal preference. But be sure that the toothpaste you choose doesn't contain flavoring agents like sugar that cause or contribute to tooth decay. All ADA-approved options don't, so if you're unsure about a toothpaste, it's best to go with one that earned the organization's Seal of Acceptance, experts say.

Yes, your toothpaste needs fluoride — here's why. (2024, May 3). NBC News. https://www.nbcnews.com/select/shopping/best-toothpastes-ncna1294664

We talked about the Sodium lauryl sulfate a little earlier. It's not going to kill us. After doing some searching, I found this.

One of the reasons you'll find it in so many different products is because it's cheap to produce, abundant, and it works well to create products that foam, lather and bubble.

What Is Sodium Lauryl Sulfate? Where It's Found and Risks - Dr. Axe. (2022, March 28). Dr. Axe. https://draxe.com/beauty/sodium-lauryl-sulfate/

Sodium Lauryl Sulfate is deemed safe. It may cause your hair loss due to follicle damage. It may cause a skin rash. But! It makes BUBBLES. It is worth noting bubbles are said to help carry away debris from cuts and wounds etc.

Do you know how they say "9 out of 10 dentists recommend" whatever toothpaste they're selling? I found the tenth dentist. What they have to say is probably worth noting.

The Studies Don't Support the Benefits of Fluoride

The scientific and medical community has spent considerable time researching and studying fluoride. Over the years, there has been very little evidence supporting the use of fluoride. That means given the results of the research studies, there is currently not enough evidence to suggest using fluoride enhanced toothpastes and mouthwashes or undergoing fluoride treatment is beneficial. Considering there is no conclusive evidence that suggests fluoride is beneficial, we believe it is best to not use it. Why put an unknown chemical component in your body if it provides no benefit to you?

Potential Health Problems that can be Linked to Ingesting Too Much Fluoride

Exposure to a tiny bit of fluoride probably won't cause harmful, lasting effects. Unfortunately, ingesting or exposing yourself to too much fluoride can cause numerous health problems. Some of the problems that have been linked to ingesting or being exposed to too much fluoride include:

Arthritis

Increased risk of bone fractures

Cancer

Brain damage

Impairment in learning

Memory problems

Neurobehavioral deficits

High blood pressure

Arterial calcification

Increased risk of heart attacks, heart failure, and strokes

Increased risk of developing peripheral arterial disease

Diabetes

Hypersensitivity

Kidney disease

Skeletal fluorosis

Thyroid disease

Issues with male fertility

Endocrine disruption

Increased risk of developing GI disorders

Avoiding fluoride can be difficult. It seems to be almost everywhere from the water you drink to toothpaste and mouthwashes. There are options available to you if you are trying to avoid fluoride, such as drinking filtered or bottled water and purchasing all-natural non-fluoride enhanced toothpaste, but it can be hard to avoid as it really is almost everywhere

Baker, J., & Baker, J. (2018, March 26). Why we Choose Not To Use Fluoride. Smiles by Shields Dentistry. https://www.smilesbyshields.com/why-we-choose-not-to-use-fluoride/

If I lived in Florida, I would be willing to be patient...

Coconut oil has been used for centuries as an effective oral hygiene practice. Current research suggests oil pulling with coconut oil (swishing oil in your mouth for 10 to 20 minutes) may reduce bad bacteria in the mouth, prevent gingivitis and tooth decay, and get rid of bad breath.

Rd, K. M. (2021, May 21). Why Coconut Oil Is Good for Your Teeth. Healthline. https://www.healthline.com/nutrition/coconut-oil-and-teeth

Get healthy and more intelligent. Reading a bit more never hurt.

I learned that our body requires 102 vitamins and minerals daily. Not just the 13 essentials.

WE DO NOT GET THEM. Most of our supplements do not come close to providing us with all of these necessities. The bare minimum is 13. I researched quite a bit on this topic. Every search that comes up is always saying the essentials. Thirteen essential vitamins. Correct. Essential. Bare minimum. Must have to function. Unfortunately, most publicly educated people weren't informed of this. I'm not surprised either. Knowing that the one who developed our school system and banking system, as well as many other systems still in place that have kept us ignorant, poor and dying was questionably quoted as saying "I don't want a nation of thinkers, I want a nation of workers." This quote has been debated. But, this one hasn't.

" THE WAY TO MAKE MONEY IS TO BUY WHEN BLOOD IS RUNNING IN THE STREETS"

John D. Rockefeller. (2024, January 2). Wikiquote. https://en.wikiquote.org/wiki/John_D._Rockefeller

Thanks a lot Dick. I mean John...

Alot of our commercial vitamins are produced with petroleum industry byproducts. I wonder why, Dick... I mean John! I'm bad with names.

Why won't our doctors tell us about or call natural remedies "medicine"? During my studies, I came across the 1910 Flexner report. This was the nail in the coffin. This was when our medical system was basically highjacked and overtaken by the elite, who were pushing what, after 115 years, I would call a very sinister motive. They removed the disadvantaged and minorities from the medical field by closing all but a few medical universities. They gained their monopoly and it basically is when "big pharma" was born.

After learning all of this, I stay as natural as I can. And it just so happens that sea moss contains 92 of the 102 vitamins and minerals our bodies need. We added our B complex with dragon fruit. Did you know we need a little bit of gold in our diet? I did not know that. Nor did I know we needed the remaining 100+ vitamins, minerals and nutrients. I

just assumed that when taking a multivitamin, it would be all of them. They're not in there. They all play such a crucial role in our lives. Did you know that gray hair can be caused by a copper deficiency? Did you know that copper also helps us stop wrinkles as it promotes our skin's elasticity by encouraging collagen absorption? Which, in turn, is keeping us looking young? Did you also know that our skin's elasticity is what keeps our veins in place and helps keep our blood circulating properly? Not only does copper deficiency cause premature gray hair. It also causes:

Fatigue and weakness

Frequent sickness

Weak and brittle bones

Problems with memory and learning

Difficulties walking

Sensitivity to cold

Pale skin

Vision Loss

Rd, R. R. M. (2023, March 21). 9 Signs and Symptoms of Copper Deficiency. Healthline. https://www.healthline.com/nutrition/copper-deficiency-symptoms

I learned this and bought a copper vessel online with some cups. I got it and made some water. Let it sit. I poured a cup, and I was instantly back on my grandpa's farm as a child. I hadn't had that taste in so long that it was a forgotten memory. He always kept these copper cups around, and I never thought much about them. Until now. So, a cup in the morning is what I drink. Don't forget, there is always too much of a good thing. Which is the reason we all have our issues in way or another. Even if it's too much of not enough. Of course, copper toxicity isn't pretty either. Always use one's best judgment and know your body as much as possible. I wish to believe all of our doctors have our best intentions in mind. I unfortunately know that may not be always the priority. This is a quote from the National Library of Medicine:

Oaths are neither a universal endeavor, nor a legal obligation, and they cannot guarantee morality. So why should doctors take an oath at all? In 1992 a BMA working party found that affirmation may strengthen a doctor's resolve to behave with integrity in extreme circumstances.

National Center for Biotechnology Information (NCBI)[Internet]. Bethesda (MD): National Library of Medicine (US), National Center for Biotechnology Information; [1988] – [cited 2024 May 18]. Available from: https://www.ncbi.nlm.nih.gov/pmc/articles/PMC1121898/

This being a fact tells us, indeed, that there is nothing but their word guaranteeing they genuinely do care. In my opinion, once again. If you have ever been in a doctor's office, then you may have had a chance to see for yourself that there is definitely no guarantee. Some are amazing. Some seem to have no care for their patients at all. If they don't. Leave.

Tell them to kiss your ass and leave. Find someone who gives a damn about you and your well-being. One that will tell you the truth.

With all degrees, you don't have to get a perfect G.P.A. to graduate. You can attain a medical degree with A's, B's, and C's.

Most medical schools in the U.S. and Canada will not accept a GPA lower than 3.0. To be competitive, students should aim for a GPA of 3.7 or higher. Schools in the Caribbean may accept a GPA as low as 2.0.

12 Ways to Get Into Med School With a Low GPA + Requirements. (n.d.). https://www.stepful.com/post/how-to-get-into-med-school-with-a-low-gpa#

Let's let that sink in. Do you have an A, B, or C Doctor? Just some questions one might contemplate. Let's head over to our "*Recipe*".

The Recipe

THIS IS NOT MEDICAL ADVICE

"It's either this or die." This seems to be their attitude toward you when they offer you chemotherapy. Being who I am, I figured that is the same attitude we need when it comes to our food. To encourage the process, it helps to have a routine. Once we established a routine, it became second nature. It didn't take much to get the kids on board. And it certainly doesn't take a lot to make time for family meals. If it's a priority, then we will make it happen. I know we tend to put other priorities before a healthy dinner with our families. We typically allow work and our daily distractions to stop us from going home and setting the table. I did. When someone you love is on their way to check out of this world, we tend to make it more of a priority to be there. I was all of a sudden able to tell people, "No, I cannot stay and work longer." I took myself home and got involved. The money it takes to eat out for a family of four at a fast-food restaurant is around $40 anymore and going up. Dine-in restaurants are $60 and up. To kill yourself with their ultra-processed, ready-made foods. (Your vegetables come out of a can and get microwaved in the dine-in fancy restaurants most of the time.) Some places are nice and coat their corn in sugar before they cook it, and most people have no idea. The kitchens are only as clean as their dirtiest cooks. And you pay top dollar for someone who won't wash their hands properly to cook your food? When I was 18 years old, I was a line cook, and we were preparing for the menu that day. There was a large group of children coming for a field trip. They all wanted ham and cheese sandwiches. I looked down the line at the thirty-something man making the sandwiches, and I joke you not. This guy was licking his fingers to separate each piece of cheese to put on the sandwiches. Don't forget. They don't use expensive cheese. It's the government made block cheese (pre-sliced, of course). I lost it. I kicked him out of the kitchen. The boss came in and watched me throw away all the food he made. She started yelling at me. Then I explained what happened, and she stormed out and kicked the guy out of the restaurant. Thankfully. The fact is, this happens all of the time, and no one is the wiser.

Now, let me ask you again. Can you still not afford to eat healthy foods at home? The most common foods we eat and the uncommon foods we pay top dollar for are killing us. Regardless of who you are, where do you eat? It is literally what you eat that does it. Two common items are loved every day by a lot of people. We discussed them earlier. Due to their having to be removed from our diets, I feel it is necessary to provide the reasoning behind it. Hot chips. Most brands are basically using the same ingredients. Just a few tweaks in chemicals here and there.

Here are a few of their ingredients and what they do:

ARTIFICIAL COLOR [RED 40 LAKE, YELLOW 6 LAKE, YELLOW 6, YELLOW 5.

FD&C RED 40 (E129) – Allure Red: This azo dye is banned in more than six European countries and was voluntarily phased out of the UK. However, it continues to be used and sold in the USA, Australia and New Zealand. It is commonly found in sports nutrition powders and can cause some serious side effects. These include dizziness, muscle pain, heart palpitations, asthma, shortness of breath, lowered libido and liver tumours.

FD&C YELLOW 6 (E110) – Sunset Yellow: This artificial colour has been banned in Norway because it's known to cause nasal congestion, hives, allergies, kidney tumors, DNA damage, hyperactivity, abdominal pain, headaches, migraines, vomiting, nausea, hormonal changes and more.

FD&C YELLOW 5 (E102) – Tartrazine: This chemical colourant is approved for use in foods in Australia, New Zealand and the USA. However, in 2010 the European Union legislated that foodstuffs containing tartrazine carry this package warning "Tartrazine may have an adverse effect on activity and attention in children." It has also been linked to asthma, migraines, thyroid cancer, weight gain, anxiety, clinical depression, blurred vision, purple skin spots and unexplainable itching.

Haglund, G. (2023, January 12). A Colourful Con - Harmful Effects of Artificial Colours. Switch Nutrition. https://switchnutrition.com.au/blogs/news/a-colourful-con-harmful-effects-of-artificial-colours#

Lakes are formed by reacting straight dyes (such as FD&C Yellow No. 5) with precipitants and salts. Aluminum may be a component. Lakes may be used as color additives for tablet coatings due to their stability. Lakes are also used in cosmetic products.

FD&C Yellow No. 5 Aluminum Lake: What is it and where is it used? (n.d.). Drugs.com. https://www.drugs.com/inactive/fd-c-yellow-no-5-aluminum-lake-323.html

Lakes, according to my research, appear in our foods and cosmetics as an aluminum-based ingredient more and more. To us, our items look very vibrant: yellow, red, blue, etc. It's in our foods, drinks, make-up, vitamins, and medications. If we consume it, they infuse it.

Lakes are technically classified as pigments, and are formed by combining a dye with a mordant, which is a metallic salt. The FDA describes lakes as: "Extensions on a substratum of alumina, of a salt prepared from one of the water-soluble straight colors by combining such colors with the basic radical aluminum calcium." The specific substrate (or "mordant") FD&C lakes utilize is alumina hydrate. This is the "metallic salt" on which the dye is precipitated or absorbed—forming a lake.

LAKE PIGMENTS - Pylam Dyes. (2023, June 30). Pylam Dyes. https://www.pylamdyes.com/colorants/lake-pigments#

Aluminum contamination of food represents an important issue to find relationships between aluminum intake and certain serious illness such as Alzheimer's disease, Parkinson's disease, dialysis encephalopathy, bone disorder, human breast cancer, and it is also considered to be a neurotoxin; aluminum salts can be accumulated by the gut and different human tissues (bones, parathyroid, and brain). Aluminum is diversely affecting the growth rate of human brain cells.

National Center for Biotechnology Information (NCBI)[Internet]. Bethesda (MD): National Library of Medicine (US), National Center for Biotechnology Information; [1988] – [cited 2024 May 18]. Available from: https://www.ncbi.nlm.nih.gov/pmc/articles/PMC6804775/#

A postmortem study of aluminum levels in various brain regions revealed that the pineal gland accumulates aluminum at a rate that is at least twice that of other brain regions. Premature infants exposed to aluminum in intravenous therapy experience neurological damage and mental impairment. A study on the neurological effects of occupational exposure to aluminum revealed sleep disturbance as a common complaint, with insomnia being reported in 22.4% of cases and sleepiness in 14.9%. A review of the underlying mechanisms of aluminum toxicity is presented in where an argument for a direct role of pineal gland disruption is developed. We do not mean to imply that pineal gland dysfunction is the only neuropathology following aluminum exposure, but we believe it plays a significant role, as sleep disorder is associated with most neurological diseases.

Seneff, S., Swanson, N., & Li, C. (2015, January 1). Aluminum and Glyphosate Can Synergistically Induce Pineal Gland Pathology: Connection to Gut Dysbiosis and Neurological Disease. Agricultural Sciences. https://doi.org/10.4236/as.2015.61005

That's just the food dye effects on our bodies from "hot chips", and other dyed foods. We know about the vanilla. At this point, is it so bad? Soy. It's always a debate. Does it hurt us? Does it help us? People have argued. I believe wars may have been started over this topic. I only joke. I think? As far as cancer is concerned and according to the National Library of Medicine: Women with breast cancer antigens (BCa) and those that are at high risk should avoid soy. We need to recall that most hereditary "traits" are just passed down bad habits and diets. These tend to create the "hereditary" conditions.

The historically low incidence rates of BCa in countries in which soy foods have been a traditional part of the diet (159) helped fuel speculation that isoflavones exert anti-estrogenic effects thereby potentially offering protection against this disease (160). However, research published beginning in the late 1990s showed that genistein (28) and isoflavone-rich SPI (161) stimulated the growth of existing ER-positive mammary tumors in ovariectomized athymic mice. In addition, in this model isoflavones inhibited the efficacy of the breast cancer drugs tamoxifen (162, 163) and letrozole (164). These findings drew attention to the ER agonistic properties of isoflavones and led to clinicians advising their BCa patients to limit or avoid soy

Let's talk about almond "milk." The side effects of your store-bought almond milk or coffee shop add-ins are not exactly healthy. There is one. I had to find the answer to end the debate. I think for the world at this point. Which substitute should you use? We never know. It turns out one is actually more beneficial. It DOESN'T SEEM TO CAUSE KIDNEY STONES IN 30–40-YEAR-OLD "HEALTHY" PEOPLE. Although...

Oat, macadamia, rice, and soy milk compare favorably in terms of kidney stone risk factors with dairy milk, whereas almond and cashew milk have more potential stone risk factors. Coconut milk may be a favorable dairy substitute for patients with chronic kidney disease based on low potassium, sodium, and oxalate.

Borin, J. F., Knight, J., Holmes, R. P., Joshi, S., Goldfarb, D. S., & Loeb, S. (2022, May 1). Plant-Based Milk Alternatives and Risk Factors for Kidney Stones and Chronic Kidney Disease. Journal of Renal Nutrition. https://doi.org/10.1053/j.jrn.2021.03.011

There you have it. Coconut milk has many amazing benefits for us.

While the majority of research and discussion surrounding the effects of coconut consumption on health have focused on cardiovascular health, there is evidence that coconut consumption may positively impact other diseases. Alzheimer's disease (AD) is a progressive neurogenerative disease and is the most common type of dementia.

I guess the coconut can maybe help fix the Alzheimer's disease we may have developed from eating, drinking, and covering our armpits in aluminum. Maybe.

Potassium Sorbate: A preservative used to suppress formation of molds and yeasts in foods, wines and personal care products. In-vitro studies suggest that it is toxic to DNA and has a negative effect on immunity.

Artificial Sweeteners: Aspartame (NutraSweet), Saccharin (Sweet N' Low), and Sucralose (Splenda) are examples of common artificial sweeteners. The original aspartame studies showed that the drug has triggered brain, mammary, uterine, ovarian, testicular, thyroid, and pancreatic tumors. More recent studies show that aspartame increases the risk of heart attack and stroke. Studies on animals have shown that saccharin can cause cancer and it is listed as a carcinogen by the World Health Organization. The U.S. Congress intervened to permit its use in the United States with a warning label. Sucralose has not been subjected to long-term health studies in humans.

These are just a few common ingredients in your everyday food chain, coffee shops, and your bag of "hot chips" and their side effects.

SUGAR: We used fresh honey to substitute for our sugar usage. Honey has more benefits than we

could imagine. It was the anti-cancer effects on our bodies for us at the time. It turns out:

The anti-tumor effects of honey have been examined using several cancer cell lines and tissue. Honey has been proven to decrease the tumorigenicity of different cancer types including breast, lung, skin, renal, prostate, colorectal, and cervical cancer. Moreover, honey has been proven to enhance the effects of chemotherapeutic drugs such as 5-fluorouracil and paclitaxel.

What Are The Health Benefits Of Honey? (2021, November 17). News-Medical. https://www.news-medical.net/health/What-Are-The-Health-Benefits-Of-Honey.aspx

We use honey in our homemade breads and teas, etc. We cut out anything that is unnatural and processed. We found that even most substitions that are used to replace sugar because it's "bad" for you are still BAD for US. Honey. Fruits. Anything with natural sugars is fine for most people. I will say it again. Know your body. Recognizing that sugar and its substitutions, like sucralose, are killing us is not the same. We try to stop using man-made foods and medicines as much as possible. It's just obvious to us at this point where most of our problems lie. Sugar alone is linked to a variety of health concerns, but the substitutes, I believe, are worse. They have shown to cause:

Increased risk of weight gain. ...

Increased cravings for sweet foods. ...

Digestive issues. ...

Negative impact on gut health. ...

Increased risk of metabolic disorders. ...

Potential impact on cardiovascular health. ...

Altered taste perception.

Potential link to cancer.

Here Are The Adverse Effects Of Consuming Artificial Sweeteners. (n.d.). NDTV.com. https://www.ndtv.com/health/here-are-the-adverse-effects-of-consuming-artificial-sweeteners-4206483

Notice that weight gain is the first side effect. Yet it's what is used in every "diet" soft drink, etc. Of course, we know that you can't spell diet without... I feel like this would be a good place for a pun.

I can see the pattern emerging from all of this, and I'm okay with not eating this literal "junk food."

WATER: If you want cleaner water in your home, I must advise you to check out Planet One Solutions as a resource.: Jeff-Louis: is more helpful than one could imagine. The water treatment plants do not remove a lot of the chemicals we put into our tap water through our own urine. You may want to know. The birth control and many other drugs and chemicals (like chemo drugs) we pass through our systems. We evacuate our body toxins to have them returned to us in our tap water. He can fix that.

Planet One Solutions – Net-Positive Solutions for Our One Planet. (n.d.). https://planetonesolutions.org/

Here's six ways to make Alkaline water at home according to wikihow.

1Add ½ to 1 tsp (3-6 g) of baking soda into 8 oz (237 mL) of water. Baking soda is a natural cooking ingredient that's also highly alkaline. With its pH of 9, it easily raises your water's pH. Simply pour ½ to 1 tsp (3-6 g) of baking soda into an 8 oz (237 mL) glass of water and stir or shake the glass well to fully combine the baking soda and water.[2]

Drink no more than 1 glass of baking soda each day. Ingesting large quantities of baking soda can be toxic and cause vomiting, diarrhea, and muscle weakness.[3]

Do not drink water alkalized with baking soda if you are on a low-sodium diet for health reasons. Baking soda is high in sodium.

2 Squeeze lemon juice into an 8 oz (237 mL) glass of water. While lemons are very acidic and have a low pH between 2 and 3, your body metabolizes them as an alkaline food. So, making lemon water might alkalize water when you drink it.[4] Simply slice or squeeze half a lemon into an 8 oz (237 mL) glass of water for a tasty, refreshing drink.[5]

Or, make a large batch of lemon water by thinly slicing 2 lemons into 2 quarts (1.9 L) of water. Chill the water in the fridge for 2 to 4 hours to give the lemons time to infuse into the water.

While lemons do cause your urine to be more alkaline, there is no clear evidence that suggests lemons alter your body's pH.

To make your lemon water more mineral-rich, add 1 tbsp (17 g) of salt.

3 Add cucumber slices into 2 quarts (1.9 L) of water. Like lemons, cucumbers are processed as an alkaline food when you eat them.[6] Making cucumber water might be a way to alkalize your water. Just chop 1 cucumber into thin slices and add them to a pitcher. Pour 2 quarts (1.9 L) of water on top and place the pitcher in the fridge for 2 to 4 hours before drinking.

4 Pour pH drops into an 8 oz (237 mL) glass of water. Alkaline are a concentrated liquid made of minerals that raise the pH levels of your water to alkalize it. Just follow the directions on your bottle of pH drops to determine how many drops to pour into a regular, 8 oz (237 mL) glass of water.[7]

While pH drops increase the alkalinity of your water, they do not filter out chemicals in your water, like chlorine or fluoride.

If you want to get rid of the impurities and chemicals in your water, use a water filter pitcher. Or, distill your own water.

5 Filter your water through an alkaline, or ionizing, water filter. An alkaline or ionizing water filter pitcher uses a mineralized filter to raise the pH levels in your water. These filters work similarly to traditional water filter pitchers, where you simply pour in the water and wait for it to pass through the filter. The series of filters in the pitcher saturate your water with alkaline minerals while also removing impurities.

6 Install a water ionizer machine. A water ionizer is a small machine that you typically attach to a faucet in your home. The machine separates your tap water into alkaline and acidic water through a process called electrolysis, where an electrical charge changes the composition of the water. While that might sound complicated, using a water ionizer is as easy as selecting how alkaline you want your water to come out of your tap.[9] Water ionizer machines are typically expensive and cost upwards of $500. If you plan to drink alkaline water often, buying an ionizer can be a more cost-effective option in the long run. Don't discard the acidic water the ionizer produces. Use it to make homemade cleaning solutions or to wash your body, as acidic water can kill bacteria.

Dietitians, F. B. (2023, December 4). How to Make Alkaline Water at Home: 6 Simple Ways. wikiHow. https://www.wikihow.com/Make-Alkaline-Water#

At first, I was hesitant to spend the money to buy a reverse osmosis system for our home. We don't necessarily have to. But after learning our lessons, I absolutely bought an R.O. system with an alkaline filter. In my opinion it is still not enough.

EPA has not determined whether standards are necessary for some drinking water contaminants, such as personal care products. Personal care products, such as cosmetics, sunscreens, and fragrances; and pharmaceuticals, including prescription, over-the-the counter, and veterinary medications, can enter water systems after use by humans or domestic animals66 and have been measured at very low levels in drinking water sources. Many concentrated animal feeding operations treat livestock with hormones and antibiotics, and can be one significant source of pharmaceuticals in water. Other major sources of pharmaceuticals in water are human waste, manufacturing plants and hospitals, and other human activities such as showering and swimming. Drinking water is a known source of lead exposure among children in the United States, particularly from corrosion of pipes and other elements of the drinking water distribution systems. Exposure to lead via drinking water may be particularly high among very young children who consume baby formula prepared with drinking water that is contaminated by leaching lead pipes. The National Toxicology Program has concluded that childhood lead exposure is associated with reduced cognitive function, reduced academic achievement, and increased attention-related behavioral problems.

Drinking Water Contaminants. (2015, October). www.epa.gov. Retrieved May 18, 2024, from https://www.epa.gov/sites/default/files/2015-10/documents/ace3_drinking_water.pdf

Something is wrong here. I can feel it.

The filtration isn't enough. The amount of aluminum consumed in drinking water is approximately 5% of the total daily intake. Thus, it is possible that some factors that prevent or accelerate aluminum absorption may exist in drinking water. We are putting different forms of aluminum in and on our bodies every day. We swipe it into our armpits with our deodorant. We eat it and drink it in almost every man-made food dye on the market. All the testing that is available on the internet says that it is safe. The FDA says it's safe. (SMCL) of 0.05–0.2 mg/L for aluminum in drinking water. The SMCL is not based on levels that will affect humans or animals. It is based on taste, smell, or color. The FDA has determined that aluminum used as food additives and Medicinal's such as antacids are generally safe. FDA set a limit for bottled water of 0.2 mg/L.

Yet, in the same paper it says:

Effects in children: Brain and bone disease caused by high levels of aluminum in the body have been seen in children with kidney disease. Bone disease has also been seen in children taking some medicines containing aluminum. In these children, the bone damage is caused by aluminum in the stomach preventing the absorption of phosphate, a chemical compound required for healthy bones. Aluminum is found in breast milk, but only a small amount of this aluminum will enter the infant's body through breastfeeding. Typical aluminum concentrations in human breast milk range from 0.0092 to 0.049 mg/L. Aluminum is also found in soy-based infant formula (0.46–0.93 mg/L) and milk-based infant formula (0.058–0.15 mg/L).

Human Oral exposure to aluminum is usually not harmful. Some studies show that people exposed to high levels of aluminum may develop Alzheimer's disease, but other studies have not found this to be true. We do not know for certain that aluminum causes Alzheimer's disease. Some people who have kidney disease store a lot of aluminum in their bodies. The kidney disease causes less aluminum to be removed from the body in the urine. Sometimes, these people developed bone or brain diseases that doctors think were caused by the excess aluminum. Although aluminum-containing over the counter oral products is considered safe in healthy individuals at recommended doses, some adverse effects have been observed following long-term use in some individuals.

PUBLIC HEALTH STATEMENT. (n.d.). CDC.gov. Retrieved May 18, 2024, from https://www.atsdr.cdc.gov/toxprofiles/tp22-c1.pdf

The doctors that study Alzheimer's disease apparently haven't been reading or keeping up with science. I found in the National Library of Medicine:

However, it is widely accepted that Aluminum is a recognized neurotoxin, and that it could cause cognitive deficiency and dementia when it enters the brain and may have various adverse effects on CNS. In general, the absorption of metals by the gastrointestinal tract is widely variable and is influenced by various factors including an individual difference, age, pH, stomach contents [173]. Recent studies using mass spectrometry of ^{26}Al have demonstrated that small, but a considerable amount of Aluminum crosses the blood brain barrier, enters into the brain, and accumulates in a semipermanent manner [174, 175]. Therefore, Aluminum can cause severe health problems in particular populations, including infants, elderly people, and patients with impaired renal functions, and unnecessary exposure to Al should be avoided for such patients [176].

National Center for Biotechnology Information (NCBI)[Internet]. Bethesda (MD): National Library of Medicine (US), National Center for Biotechnology Information; [1988] – [cited 2024 May 18]. Available from: https://www.ncbi.nlm.nih.gov/pmc/articles/PMC3056430/

An abstract suggesting that women are at an increased risk for breast cancer due to the aluminum in their anti-perspirants: Since aluminium (Al) pervades our environment, the scientific community has for many years raised concerns regarding its safety in humans. Al is present in numerous cosmetics such as antiperspirants, lipsticks and sunscreens. Al chlorohydrate is the active antiperspirant agent in underarm cosmetics and may constitute for Al a key exposure route to the human body and a potential source of damage. An in vitro study has demonstrated that Al from antiperspirant can be absorbed through viable human stripped skin. The potential toxicity of Al has been clearly shown and recent works convincingly argue that Al could be involved in cancerogenic processes. Nowadays, for example, Al is suspected of being involved in breast cancer. Recent work in cells in culture has lent credence to the hypothesis that this metal could accumulate in the mammary gland and selectively interfere with the biological properties of breast epithelial cells, thereby promoting a cascade of alterations reminiscent of the early phases of malignant transformation. In addition, several studies suggest that the presence of Al in human breast could influence metastatic process. As a consequence, given that the toxicity of Al has been widely recognized and that it is not a physiological component in human tissues, reducing the concentration of this metal in antiperspirants is a matter of urgency.

National Center for Biotechnology Information (NCBI)[Internet]. Bethesda (MD): National Library of Medicine (US), National Center for Biotechnology Information; [1988] – [cited 2024 May 18]. Available from: https://pubmed.ncbi.nlm.nih.gov/24418462/

The arguments have been that we are supposed to pass the majority of the aluminum and metals we consume, through our bodies when we use the restroom. Only a small trace amount stays, and an

even smaller amount settles in our brains. Unless our kidneys are not fully functioning due to overconsumption of all of these other "poisons". Then it goes straight to our brains. Assuming our kidneys are fully functional, over time that small "safe to consume" amount builds up. The rate of its buildup depends on the consumer. In the end, the aluminum is settling in our brains and causing our neurological disorders as elderly people. It may be settling in and causing breast cancer. None of this apparently matters to the powers that be. I found this article and because they tested them for six whole months, I am here to let you know that it is okay and now all is well. Nothing to see here...

A 6-MONTH DIETARY TOXICITY STUDY OF ACIDIC SODIUM ALUMINIUM PHOSPHATE IN BEAGLE DOGS:

dietary administration of sodium aluminum phosphate for 6 months at concentrations of 3% or lower caused no significant toxicological effects in beagle dogs.

Katz, A., Frank, D., Sauerhoff, M., Zwicker, G., & Freudenthal, R. (1984, January 1). *A 6-month dietary toxicity study of acidic sodium aluminium phosphate in beagle dogs*. Food and Chemical Toxicology. https://doi.org/10.1016/0278-6915(84)90045-0

The dogs made it! As for us...

We tend to carry metals in our bodies, apparently, in small amounts until we are old and have the added bonus of forgetting everything. We get a little dose of aluminum with the fluoride in our water, among the many other chemicals they allow. Although fluoride is used industrially in a fluorine compound, the manufacture of ceramics, pesticides, aerosol propellants, refrigerants, glassware, and Teflon cookware, it is a generally unwanted byproduct of aluminium, fertilizer, and iron ore manufacture.

National Center for Biotechnology Information (NCBI)[Internet]. Bethesda (MD): National Library of Medicine (US), National Center for Biotechnology Information; [1988] – [cited 2024 May 18]. Available from: https://www.ncbi.nlm.nih.gov/pmc/articles/PMC3956646/#

Do you think they mass produce the one they have to dig for? Or is it the one that's already available from the recycling centers?

Our toothpaste is full of it. Most people don't realize that it took a lawsuit to get the government to release the actual findings of fluoride effects on our bodies.

Around 210 million Americans today have access to artificially fluoridated tap water, and the policy has had a pronounced effect on oral health by reducing tooth decay. It's widely hailed as a public health success story. In the current lawsuit, plaintiffs are taking a long-standing and, to many experts, provocative stance, arguing that water fluoridation poses a risk to human health, and that the Environmental Protection Agency is obligated to address the issue. The outcome of the case could effectively end water fluoridation in United States. A ruling from Judge Edward M. Chen is expected soon.

Schulson, M. (2024, March 6). Baring Teeth: The Long Battle Over Fluoride Comes to a Head. Undark Magazine. https://undark.org/2024/03/06/fluoride-drinking-water/#

This is concerning.

Although fluoride is used industrially in a fluorine compound, the manufacture of ceramics, pesticides, aerosol propellants, refrigerants, glassware, and Teflon cookware, it is a generally unwanted byproduct of aluminium, fertilizer, and iron ore manufacture.

The inability to control individual dose renders the notion of an "optimum concentration" obsolete. in the USA, a study in Iowa found that 90% of 3-month-olds consumed over their recommended upper limits, with some babies ingesting over 6 mg of fluoride daily, above what the Environmental Protection Agency and the WHO say is safe to avoid crippling skeletal fluorosis [41]. Second, all nutrient values for fluoride need to be withdrawn, not least because it is irrational to have daily nutrient intakes for a hazardous substance whose mode of action is topical on teeth enamel. Third, coordinated global efforts to reduce adverse human health effects on fluoride need to start with ensuring that its introduction into water supplies is prohibited, occupational and industrial fluoride exposures and injuries are reduced to the minimum possible, and natural water systems with high fluoride content are defluoridated prior to being endorsed as "potable." Finally, given that dental caries is the most common disease globally arising from bacterial infection [91, 92], efforts to develop safe technologies to address the disease deserve high priority. Unfortunately, advocacy for funding to develop nonfluoride approaches for dental caries prevention has so far been compromised by the "religious arguments" between antifluoridationists and profluoridationists.

National Center for Biotechnology Information (NCBI)[Internet]. Bethesda (MD): National Library of Medicine (US), National Center for Biotechnology Information; [1988] – [cited 2024 May 18]. Available from: https://www.ncbi.nlm.nih.gov/pmc/articles/PMC3956646/

Filter your water, folks. To make alkaline water, we would take two lemons and cut them up, toss them in the pitcher, fill it with water, let it sit overnight in the fridge, and you would have naturally alkaline water. We drank at the very least, a glass a day. I add in cucumber as well. In addition to the "normal" water. I have found that we as people don't like normal water. It lacks consistency and sugars that we have been conditioned to drink, i.e., soda and energy drinks etc. This did help us stop drinking all of the garbage.

BREAD: First of all, I cannot begin this portion without acknowledging Dr. Ava Nirvana, CEO, MD, NP, PHD, and MASTER FOODOLOGIST. She has many helpful recipes on her page as well as more information on our health. I agree with her opinion on quite a few topics. Go check out her page and gain some more of that delicious perspective.

Gluten Kills - Pura VIda Foodology. (2024, February 20). Pura VIda Foodology. https://dravatarnirvana.com/gluten-kills/

Now with what we know about gluten if you went and read her page. We must choose wisely. Now if you are not ready to go full gluten free. Although one should. Then we must discuss Unleavened breads. No yeast. Whole grains. Flat breads and tortillas, etc. Here is a link that lists what "good" breads may be used to replace the "bad" breads.

Sugar and Cancer. (n.d.). UCSF Osher Center for Integrative Health. https://osher.ucsf.edu/patient-care/integrative-medicine-resources/cancer-and-nutrition/faq/sugar-and-cancer

The flat breads help to remove free radicals from our systems. They contain all the same vitamins, which are high in B vitamin complex, by the way. The yeast, I believe, makes it worse in our bodies. From the alcohols we consume to the breads we eat. My example for this is: I was in high school. I had a little scratch in my throat and wasn't feeling great. I was also young and dumb. In high school, I tried to get out of my house every chance I could. I went to a friend's house, and there were a few of us there. We pooled money and got some beers. I drank two beers, and my throat started swelling. I called my mom to take me home. In my house, you literally had to be dying to go to the E.R. This was Friday. I was still breathing. Barely. Monday came. I survived the weekend on ibuprofen. At the doctor, I tested positive for mono. The doctor asked me what I had been doing. I explained what happened Friday. He told me that I most likely exacerbated the minor strep throat I had by drinking the beer, and it morphed into mono. Had I been drinking whiskey. It wouldn't have been so bad. The yeast made it worse. Now that didn't help as an adult because I used the old excuse to drink whiskey when I got sick. It didn't kill me and it didn't make it worse either. Yeast. Is not our friend in those times. I have also learned that, in nature, a lot of our foods tend to resemble our internal organs. When this occurs, the fruit or vegetable that resembles one of our organs tends to be what helps. For example. The citrus fruits like oranges and limes resemble our kidneys. They also help heal our kidney function.

Sea moss looks like our nervous system when dried and laid out. It just so happens to help heal our nerves, as well as reduce inflammation and pain affecting the nerves and joints.

Mushrooms: More wonderful still, the basic reproductive structure of a fungus, the mycelium, involves a paradigm that can be observed throughout the universe. Its network-like design mirrors that of dark matter, neural connections in the brain, and even the human-created internet

Luce. (2018, June 6). If Mushrooms Could Talk. University of Illinois Urbana-Champaign. Retrieved May 18, 2024, from https://q.sustainability.illinois.edu/a-fungal-estrangement/#

Mycelium happens to help nourish our brain's functionality. Mushrooms help clear brain fog and have many other benefits. We also have quite a debate about apricot kernels and their effects. Recently, a man named Jason Vale was arrested for a crime involving selling the seeds as a cure for

cancer. But Vale also pointed to the power of apricot seeds as the reason he survived cancer — a story he told on his website, Apricots from God, where he sold the seeds to other cancer patients for $18.95 a pound.

And that's how the arm wrestler ended up in prison.

Flynn, M. (2019, October 24). New York arm-wrestling legend and his mom arrested for selling 'Apricots From God' as bogus cancer cure. Washington Post. https://www.washingtonpost.com/nation/2019/10/24/jason-vale-apricot-seeds-cancer-cure-arrest-arm-wrestling/#

Yet, here we have directly from the National Library of Medicine.

Amygdalin from Apricot Kernels Induces Apoptosis and Causes Cell Cycle Arrest in Cancer Cells

The current review epitomizes published information and provides complete interpretations about all known anti-cancer mechanisms of amygdalin, possible role of naturally occurring amygdalin in fight against cancer and mistaken belief about cyanide toxicity causing potential of amygdalin.

National Center for Biotechnology Information (NCBI)[Internet]. Bethesda (MD): National Library of Medicine (US), National Center for Biotechnology Information; [1988] – [cited 2024 May 18]. Available from: https://pubmed.ncbi.nlm.nih.gov/29308747/

Once again. THIS IS NOT MEDICAL ADVICE. From what I have gathered in my research, there is a higher power at play in our lives that may be dictating how we are treated for our health concerns and what information we are allowed to have and share. As well as how we share it. That is merely my opinion. Now! Let's move on to our ingredients at mealtime.

BREAKFAST

Sea moss capsules 2 a day

Fenugreek capsules 1 a day

16oz frozen fruit mix banana, mango, papaya, matcha tea and then added frozen red dragon fruit

8oz grape juice

8oz apple juice

6-8 apricot kernels

Blend well. Enjoy still every morning.

When it comes to cancer-fighting foods, you can't beat the power of produce and plant-based foods. Certain fruits, vegetables, nuts, beans, oats, whole grains, spices and teas provide unique benefits not found in other foods. These benefits help reduce the risks of certain cancers and can even slow tumor growth and recurrence.

Your Seasonal Guide to Cancer-Fighting Foods - Health & Wellness | Loma Linda University Health. (n.d.). https://lluh.org/patients-visitors/health-wellness/blog/your-seasonal-guide-cancer-fighting-foods#

If certain types of cancer run in your family, you may want to start eating slightly green bananas. That's because the resistant starch in unripe bananas can reduce the risk of some cancers by more than 60 percent, according to a 20-year international study.

(2022, September 7). Cancer Study Proves Eating Unripe Bananas Has Benefits. FCP Live-In. https://www.liveinhomecare.com/cancer-study-proves-eating-unripe-bananas-has-benefits/cancer/#

The vibrant red-fleshed dragon fruit contains lycopene, a powerful antioxidant known for its heart-protective properties and potential to reduce the risk of certain cancers.

Toshi, N. (2024, May 3). 10 Health Benefits And Recipes Of Dragon Fruit (Pitaya). PharmEasy Blog. https://pharmeasy.in/blog/10-health-benefits-and-recipes-of-dragon-fruit-pitaya/#

Matcha green tea (MGT) inhibits the propagation of cancer stem cells.

National Center for Biotechnology Information (NCBI)[Internet]. Bethesda (MD): National Library of Medicine (US), National Center for Biotechnology Information; [1988] – [cited 2024 May 18]. Available from: https://www.ncbi.nlm.nih.gov/pmc/articles/PMC6128439/#

Lunch

We fasted through lunch most days with lemon water. According to Yoshinori Ohsumi, "When a person's body is hungry, he eats himself or cleans himself." Scientists have found that when a human body is exposed to hunger for not less than 8 hours and not more than 16 hours in a day, it produces special proteins called autophagosomes in all parts of the body, and they are more like giant brooms that collect around dead, cancerous, and diseased cells and analyze them and return them like an image that the body benefits from. The study advised the practice of hunger and thirst two to three times a week. In 2016, he was awarded the Nobel Prize in Physiology or Medicine "for his discoveries of mechanisms for autophagy."

National Center for Biotechnology Information (NCBI)[Internet]. Bethesda (MD): National Library of Medicine (US), National Center for Biotechnology Information; [1988] – [cited 2024 May 18]. Available from:
https://www.ncbi.nlm.nih.gov/pmc/articles/PMC3328387/

Kotifani, A. (2020, June 2). Fasting for Health and Longevity: Nobel Prize Winning Research on Cell Aging. Blue Zones. https://www.bluezones.com/2018/10/fasting-for-health-and-longevity-nobel-prize-winning-research-on-cell-aging/

When we ate, it consisted of flat breads and tortillas. Avocado spreads. We stopped eating peanut butter and soy-based everything. Avoiding foods that mess with our body's natural balance of hormones has been proven to reduce a plethora of health concerns and issues for men and women alike. Including, but not limited to:

Male pattern baldness and thinning hair

Loss of facial firmness

Gynecomastia (man boobs)

Abdominal obesity (belly fat)

Decreased libido

Loss of muscle mass and strength

Increased body fat

Mood changes (irritability, depression, anxiety)

Difficulty concentrating, memory problems, and mental fog

Insomnia

Lack of motivation and drive

Hot flashes

Loss of self confidence

McAvennie, M. (2024, March 4). Avoid These 11 Testosterone Killing Foods. Hone Health. https://honehealth.com/edge/nutrition/foods-that-lower-testosterone/

Dinner

Typically consisted of protein, "good starch", cayenne pepper in some form or another, vegetable, fruit. Among many cancer-fighting beneficial herbs and spices is cayenne pepper. It is easy to incorporate into dinner meals. As well as turmeric, ginger, saffron and oregano all contain cancer fighting properties. The cayenne pepper helps us lose weight at the same time it helps fight cancer.

Cayenne Pepper: This hot pepper contains capsaicin, a powerful antioxidant that helps with weight loss and is an anti-inflammatory food. Cayenne also contains beta-carotene. It is known to be toxic to cancer cells and helps prevent growth of cancer cells.

Video With Transcript. (n.d.). Website. https://www.mhs.net/news/2016/09/cancer-fighting-herbs-and-spices#

Onions have many benefits for us as well. Popular around the world, onions are celebrated for their strong antibacterial, anti-parasitic, and less likely antifungal properties. In a study conducted by Ebrahimi et al. [37], it was shown that onion extracts had a more potent antibacterial effect against *Streptococcus mutans* than *Streptococcus sanguinis*. The antibacterial activity of red onions was more pronounced than yellow and green onions, respectively. As the concentration of the onions increased, the antibacterial activity also increased.

National Center for Biotechnology Information (NCBI)[Internet]. Bethesda (MD): National Library of Medicine (US), National Center for Biotechnology Information; [1988] – [cited 2024 May 18]. Available from: https://www.ncbi.nlm.nih.gov/pmc/articles/PMC10241316/#

Our original, normal dinners consisted of a 4 to 5 day a week, red meat dinner of some sorts. Does Bison meat possess anticancer nutrients? Based upon the lipid analysis of range fed Bison meat, we might predict that it might have favorable cardiovascular benefits compared to other types of meat products. Other attributes of Bison meat related to other chronic disease conditions may also exist. Cancer has recently "dethroned" heart disease as the top killer among Americans under the age of 85. If Bison meat is more "heart healthy" than other red meats, could it also possess anti-carcinogenic properties? Although this is largely conjecture since experimental evidence is lacking, there may be additional health related benefits related to the composition of Bison meat. Could the fatty acid profile of Bison (and perhaps other wild ruminant species) contribute to a reduced risk against certain types of cancer? The increased content omega 3-fatty acids and of certain beneficial C-18 unsaturated fatty acids such as conjugated linoleic acid (CLA isomers, 18:2 cis-9, trans-11 and 18:2 cis-12, trans-10) as well as the reduced content of potentially carcinogenic fatty acids such as linoleic acid (C-18:2 cis 9,12) may contribute to important nutritional properties of Bison meat (Cordain et al 2002, Rule et al 2002). CLA is believed to be a "beneficial" fatty acid, with anti-inflammatory and possibly anti-carcinogenic properties.

E.W. Askew, Ph.D. Professor, Division of Nutrition, College of Health, Health Sciences, University of Utah, Salt Lake City, Utah. (2020, February). Bison - A "Healthy" Red Meat?? National Buffalo Foundation. Retrieved May 18, 2024, from https://www.nationalbuffalofoundation.org/wp-content/uploads/2020/02/University-of-Utah-Bison-Lipid-Study.pdf

I have to take time to note a conversation with Dr. Ava. She explained to me that when we eat the meat of a larger animal, we get more of an influx from their hormones. This being due to the fact that

larger animals have larger organs. Therefore, more hormones are produced. When we eat them. We get a large 1200 lb. cow's massive influx of hormones. So, for the argument of "plants like soy give us estrogen". Yes. In very small plant dosage. Not large mammal dosages. Taking what she said and knowing that when the animals are fearful when they are slaughtered, they release another influx of chemicals into the meat. I once again agreed with her facts. So does the science...

Effect of stress during slaughter on carcass characteristics and meat quality in tropical beef cattle

National Center for Biotechnology Information (NCBI)[Internet]. Bethesda (MD): National Library of Medicine (US), National Center for Biotechnology Information; [1988] – [cited 2024 May 18]. Available from:
https://www.ncbi.nlm.nih.gov/pmc/articles/PMC7463084/

Commercial chicken leads to impaired hormone levels. The normal production is affected that causes several physical issues. For example, hypogonadism, low testosterone levels and testicular atrophy are common. Females are likely to suffer from imbalances in estrogen and progesterone levels

blog - LA ROSA Chicken & Grill. (n.d.). LA ROSA Chicken & Grill.
https://larosachicken.com/Steroids-and-Growth-Hormone-in-Chicken-Why-You-Must-Avoid-them#

These all being lessons we learned along the way and are still adjusting our menu accordingly. We flip-flopped everything. We would still have red meat dinners. Only a couple of nights a week. The red meat we would eat was either grass-fed beef that has minimal interference from man, as well as free-range bison, chicken and salmon. Then, five nights a week, we tried to have white meat. The whole intent was to keep the body's system more alkaline to inhibit cancer growth and kill it. We would add in recipes found online to help give direction. Vegetables. Fresh. As often as possible. Fruits. Fresh. As often as possible. Need a snack? Grab a piece of fruit or a vegetable. Snack on tomato and cucumber. It's not difficult to look for and find these items in your fridge if that's what you start buying. Stop buying the sugary, murder-me foods. It isn't fun in the beginning, but you can typically find your substitutes. I have found an exchange for the other when it comes to "junk' food vs. "health" food. Switched from potato chips to apple chips or banana chips. I switched from soft drinks to (this was the hardest, I believe) tea at first. Then I switched to cucumber lemon water. Then I switched to different waters. Then I discovered the oxygenated water. That helped more for me. I read an interesting piece once that said my body would be lacking calcium due to <u>when</u> I was born. I love to eat limes. Most likely, my body knows I need more calcium added to my diet, and we do happen to get amazing benefits from limes. One of those is calcium citrate. Which, we need. Research on why pirates used to need to eat limes. It's a fun fact for the water cooler. The more we learn about our bodies and what we need as individuals, the more we can make honest, health-conscious decisions in our daily routines. And these decisions will greatly increase the length and value of our time here.

I understand I am hardheaded. I don't like to follow these online guides to eating because they never quite feel right. That is because they were not written for us. They were written for the person writing them. Instead of finding a flaw in one person's process and giving up, I tried to just find one item in all of the different guides that I could relate to and incorporate into our diet. Something that I knew would benefit us and not change the entire dynamic of our meal system all at once. Every night, our family makes sure to sit down at the dinner table. We always talk about our days or address family concerns. Changing the entire dynamic would have upset the balance in the harmony of our meals. So, we just added in a little here and there. Achieving a better result that was easier for us all to adapt to. Do we miss some of the foods we ate? Yes. But was the answer honest? These "foods" were killing us. Yes. Do I prefer instant gratification? Not when it involves the length of my life. I'd like to see it play out slowly. Day by day. Not: "That's all, folks!" From one day to the next, then it's over. No, thank you. Burn out? Fade away? Maybe another option is available. Live long and prosper. I like that. Brown, S., & Brown, S. (2024, April 16). Alkalizing Meal Ideas. Alkaline for Life. https://alkalineforlife.com/blogs/news/7-days-of-alkaline-eating-ideas

Once we were healthier and felt on top of our game, we began using a tincture of wormwood, black walnut hull, and cloves. One week on and one week off. Twice. I believe this was the final process that completed the job and brought tumor down to zero. ONCE AGAIN! This is only my opinion and her results. Remember, wormwood is anti-cancer. Black walnut hull is anti-cancer. Cloves are as well, but their main function in this concoction for us was to eliminate the mucous sack the cancer hides in. This was just my logical process for addressing our plan of attack. From all the resources I had gathered

across the web, And she's still here, ladies and gentlemen.

DETOXIFICATION: While we are attacking these parasites, we must cleanse ourselves to remove the waste from our system. We used a couple of different methods. Fenugreek is known for its anti-cancer effects on breast cancer and as a powerful antioxidant. As well as increasing our natural collagen production, it also has enormous benefits that far exceed what I expected for men and women.

Fenugreek seeds are packed with essential nutrients such as fiber, iron, magnesium, and manganese, and are a rich source of phytoestrogens, which are compounds that mimic the effects of estrogen in the body. Here are some of the potential benefits of fenugreek seeds for females:

Enhances breast milk production: Fenugreek seeds have been traditionally used to promote lactation in breastfeeding mothers. Studies suggest that the galactagogue properties of fenugreek may help increase milk production.

Regulates menstrual cycle: Fenugreek seeds contain diosgenin, a compound that can help regulate menstrual cycles and relieve menstrual cramps.

Reduces menopausal symptoms: The phytoestrogens in fenugreek seeds can help alleviate hot flashes, mood swings, and other menopausal symptoms.

Improves fertility: Fenugreek seeds have been shown to improve ovarian function and increase fertility in women with polycystic ovary syndrome (PCOS).

Promotes skin health: Fenugreek seeds are a rich source of antioxidants that can help protect the skin from damage and promote healthy, glowing skin.

Toshi, N. (2024, May 6). Fenugreek (Methi) Seeds: Incredible Health and Beauty Benefits. PharmEasy Blog. https://pharmeasy.in/blog/incredible-health-and-beauty-benefits-of-fenugreek-seeds/

HONEY: Traditionally, honey is used in the treatment of eye diseases, bronchial asthma, throat infections, tuberculosis, thirst, hiccups, fatigue, dizziness, hepatitis, constipation, worm infestation, piles, eczema, healing of ulcers, and wounds and used as a nutritious supplement. The ingredients of honey have been reported to exert antioxidant, antimicrobial, anti-inflammatory, antiproliferative, anticancer, and antimetastatic effects. Many evidences suggest the use of honey in the control and treatment of wounds, diabetes mellitus, cancer, asthma, and also cardiovascular, neurological, and gastrointestinal diseases. Honey has a potential therapeutic role in the treatment of disease by phytochemical, anti-inflammatory, antimicrobial, and antioxidant properties. Flavonoids and polyphenols, which act as antioxidants, are two main bioactive molecules present in honey. According to modern scientific literature, honey may be useful and has protective effects for the treatment of various disease conditions such as diabetes mellitus, respiratory, gastrointestinal, cardiovascular, and nervous systems, even it is useful in cancer treatment because many types of antioxidants are present in honey. In conclusion, honey could be considered as a natural therapeutic agent for various medicinal purposes. Sufficient evidence exists recommending the use of honey in the management of disease conditions. Based on these facts, the use of honey in clinical wards is highly recommended.

National Center for Biotechnology Information (NCBI)[Internet]. Bethesda (MD): National Library of Medicine (US), National Center for Biotechnology Information; [1988] – [cited 2024 May 18]. Available from: https://www.ncbi.nlm.nih.gov/pmc/articles/PMC5424551/#

CHLOROPHYLL: H3O... maybe what the doctor ordered?

Chlorophyll has antioxidant properties and therefore can help to reduce damage from free radicals," says Hadley King, MD, a board-certified dermatologist specializing in medical and cosmetic dermatology. "This can make it a part of an anti-aging regimen and could improve signs of skin aging."

Clark, C., & Clark, C. (2023, August 16). Chlorophyll Is the Anti-Aging, Anti-Inflammatory Ingredient Your Skin-Care Routine Is Missing. Well+Good. https://www.wellandgood.com/chrolophyll-for-skin/#

As well as a very long list of benefits, it has also been shown to help with neurological disorders such as Alzheimer's, and here's a link for you.

National Center for Biotechnology Information (NCBI)[Internet]. Bethesda (MD): National Library of Medicine (US), National Center for Biotechnology Information; [1988] – [cited 2024 May 18]. Available from: https://www.ncbi.nlm.nih.gov/pmc/articles/PMC8225186/

EXERCISE: Please understand that we need healthy fats in our diet. Our body fat, on the other hand, is not only hard on our bodies. It is a common breeding ground for tumors. Through diet and exercise, we can eliminate the fertile ground we provide some of these cancers with. "This is the seed-and-soil hypothesis," White says. "Tumor cells like to go to places where there is fertile soil. Based on our results, we think that adipose tissue can be very fertile soil for melanoma." According to a new study by researchers at the Sloan Kettering Institute (SKI) at Memorial Sloan Kettering (MSK), melanomas prefer to grow near adipose (fat) tissue. The team, led by Richard White, a physician-scientist in the Cancer Biology and Genetics Program at SKI, showed that melanomas actively take in lipids if given the chance, and they tend to migrate toward tissues rich in fat cells.

Tontonoz, M. (n.d.). Cancer's Hidden Helper: Your Fat. Scientific American. https://www.scientificamerican.com/custom-media/cancers-hidden-helper-your-fat/#

Any kind of active movement will elevate the heart rate if it's been a while. I do get at least 90 minutes of exercise, three times a week, as a minimum. WALKING DOES NOT ELEVATE YOUR HEART RATE ENOUGH. What do I know? You have to get your blood flowing and your body moving. Too many people lie to themselves, thinking that walking is going to get our bodies burning fat and calories. It is not enough, once you've become out of shape. You have got to get moving. Start with a walk. Just don't keep walking. Speed it up every day if possible. Body fat is one problem we can kind of *run* away from, in a sense. Remember that our calf muscles act as a secondary pump to return our blood back to our hearts. If the calf muscles are too weak to deliver the blood back up, you will eventually have another kind of life-threatening health concern if you don't already. We must have our bodies fully functioning again. The good news is that it goes hand in hand with getting healthy. We get more energy. We get a better attitude toward ourselves. We feel younger and more vibrant. There is nothing wrong with being a bit "selfish" and loving ourselves. We have to start with ourselves. Or we can never truly love anything else. We must fill our cups with knowledge and thirst for more.

Crazy stuff, huh? The dyes in the food we eat and drink. The aluminum our food gets served in. The plastic it gets cooked in. The non-stick coatings of our pans. All of these have been moved out of our homes. It was not a quick, simple task. It was not difficult, though, once we saw how our health is not taken into consideration by the people who say they are in charge of our health. And when you stop spending the massive amounts of money for all of the fast-food industry to poison you, you can then afford to spend that money on better pans to cook with. I also installed a fairly inexpensive 6-filter reverse osmosis system with an alkaline filter for less than $250 off of an auction site. I also made my own alkaline water following the instructions linked. After three months, we started doing a parasite cleanse and began attacking this. The mixture of cloves, black walnut hull, and wormwood was, in my opinion, the perfect option to finish the job. Once we had gotten healthy with sea moss and dragon fruit and all of the dietary changes made, we then stayed with the routine. We added in fenugreek to help flush out toxins, and I have to point out, that I think of all the effects of every substance on the planet. Fenugreek has the most intriguing effect on our bodies. Check it out. When you sweat. You smell a hint of maple. Not B.O. It's the strangest occurrence when you're working and forget.

Castor oil is a multi-use tool for our bodies. Castor oil therapy stimulates the circulatory system. By increasing circulation, fresh oxygenated blood flows through the abdomen and pelvis and nourishes the reproductive organs, ovaries, fallopian tubes, and uterus, helping them to properly function. A lack of circulation to these organs prevents them from properly healing if damaged and may promote the formation of excessive scar tissue and adhesions.

Additional therapies like acupuncture and Chinese medicine can greatly optimize circulation and are a beneficial way to naturally support egg health and healthy reproductive organ function.

Castor Oil Therapy | Harmony Health. (2017, May 4). Harmony Health Acupuncture. https://www.harmonyhealthchicago.com/fertile-harmony/castor-oil-therapy/

Although many claim castor oil helps us by helping to remove many, in my opinion, major causes of cancer. The doctors still tell us it doesn't help us with our cancer. Regardless. I still read that and many other articles one night and woke up telling my wife that we might want to try this. She read what I read and agreed.

I had a small cyst on my wrist, and since I was doing and taking whatever she was, I of course applied a castor oil pack to my wrist daily, and it indeed disappeared. Does it work for cancer? I cannot say. We still applied packs to her stomach as well. Just in case...

After five months they scanned her again. This time. The tumor was gone. 0mm and my wife was becoming herself again. A few months later she had been screened again and there were still no signs of infection. I remember the doctor saying to her, "Whatever you're doing, keep it up."
Definitely will do doc. Will do indeed.

Extra Sauce

Let us continue, shall we? This is still not medical advice.

PARASITES CAUSE CERTAIN FORMS OF CANCER.

We are finding more and more that parasites are behind most of our ailments.

Parasites and malignancies, a review, with emphasis on digestive cancer induced by *Cryptosporidium parvum* The International Agency for Research on Cancer (IARC) identifies ten infectious agents (viruses, bacteria, and parasites) able to induce cancer disease in humans. Among parasites, a carcinogenic role is currently recognized for the digenetic trematodes *Schistosoma haematobium*, leading to bladder cancer, and *Clonorchis sinensis* or *Opisthorchis viverrini*, which cause cholangiocarcinoma. Furthermore, several reports suspected the potential association of other parasitic infections (due to protozoan or metazoan parasites) with the development of neoplastic changes in the host tissues. The present work briefly reviewed available data on the involvement of parasites in neoplastic processes in humans or animals and especially

focused on the carcinogenic power of *Cryptosporidium parvum* infection. On the whole, infection seems to play a crucial role in the etiology of cancer.

National Center for Biotechnology Information (NCBI)[Internet]. Bethesda (MD): National Library of Medicine (US), National Center for Biotechnology Information; [1988] – [cited 2024 May 18]. Available from: https://www.ncbi.nlm.nih.gov/pmc/articles/PMC3671432/

According to an article from healthline.com:

Ashpari, Z. (2023, October 20). Tips for Limiting Acidic Foods. Healthline. https://www.healthline.com/nutrition/acidic-foods#high-acid-food-and-drink

Foods considered acidic generally have a pH level of 4.6 or lower.

But the pH of food before you eat it is less important than the amount of acid or alkaline produced with digestion and metabolism of that food.

Excessive phosphorus and proteins over a long period of time can contribute to the development of metabolic acidosis. The U.S. Department of Health and Human Services recommends that protein should be 10-30%Trusted Source of your total calories.

Foods that tend to cause more acidity in the body if consumed chronically and in excess include Trusted Source:

certain dairy products, including cheese

fish and seafood

high sodium processed foods

fresh meats and processed meats, such as corned beef and turkey

certain starchy foods, such as brown rice, oat flakes, or granola

carbonated beverages, such as soda, seltzer, or spritzers

high protein foods and supplements with animal protein

National Center for Biotechnology Information (NCBI)[Internet]. Bethesda (MD): National Library of Medicine (US), National Center for Biotechnology Information; [1988] – [cited 2024 May 18]. Available from: https://www.ncbi.nlm.nih.gov/pmc/articles/PMC5490517/

In general, fruits and vegetables are more alkalizing. Including them in a diverse diet full of fruits and vegetables will help prevent the overconsumption of animal protein and the risk of developing metabolic acidosis.

Oxygen. An oxygenated environment proves inhospitable to cancer. The way to achieve that is by oxygenating your water. Go to the oxygen bars. Find a hyperbaric chamber. There are options out there. "Giving cancer cells extra oxygen might shut them down or even kill them."

Staff, D. F. (2019, November 26). Cancer and Oxygen: What’s the Connection? Dana-Farber Cancer Institute. https://blog.dana-farber.org/insight/2019/11/cancer-and-oxygen-whats-the-connection/#

Vitamin B17 kills cancer. It causes cell death in cancer. According to the national health institute. Amygdalin (Vitamin B-17) is a naturally occurring vitamin found in the seeds of the fruits of Prunus Rosacea family including apricot, bitter almond, cherry, and peach. National Center for Biotechnology Information (NCBI)[Internet]. Bethesda (MD): National Library of Medicine (US), National Center for Biotechnology Information; [1988] – [cited 2024 May 18]. Available from: https://pubmed.ncbi.nlm.nih.gov/31958042/

"Cancer cells tend to become more aggressive as they adapt to low oxygen levels,"

Mone, A., & Mehl, V. (2019, November 7). *Oxygen-Starved Tumor Cells Have Survival Advantage That Promotes Cancer Spread*. Johns Hopkins Medicine. https://www.hopkinsmedicine.org/news/newsroom/news-releases/2019/11/oxygen-starved-tumor-cells-have-survival-advantage-that-promotes-cancer-spread

The Juice

DEFINITELY NOT MEDICAL ADVICE

With most subjects, this one can be quite controversial. We find there is always some form of gaslighting or duality of opinion. Some form of contradiction seems to exist for almost every path of healing: self-discovery, logic, religion, etc. I believe in a collective consciousness. Sure. But I do not believe every person on the planet functions the same. Nor do they have the same nutritional requirements. Therefore, they would all need their own personal approach to their health and nutritional requirements.

If you have access to your medical records, then you should always know where your body is and what it may need. If not. Ask your doctor to do a blood test for any deficiencies you may have. Find yourself. As you are an individual, you deserve your own individual health plan and approach to life. Know where your bloodlines come from. What foods did the people of those regions eat? If you have an unrelenting feeling that something is wrong or cannot seem to just get healthy, then maybe take a look at what your ancestors ate.

This ready-made life has provided everyone with a very general availability of nutrition and even more supplements. Typically, it is man-made and poisonous. Even the vitamins we take. We think they come from a healthy source. But our vitamin C is derived from mold.

The first cup of fresh orange juice in the morning is not always what you think it is.

Citric acid as a food additive is not natural citric acid; it is manufactured through fermentation using *Aspergillus niger*. *Aspergillus niger* is a potent allergen. Food additive manufactured citric acid may be causing allergic inflammatory cascades. Manufactured citric acid may be contributing to the inflammation seen in asthma, juvenile idiopathic arthritis, autistic spectrum disorder, and fibromyalgia. The safety of manufactured citric acid has never been studied since it was granted GRAS status.

National Center for Biotechnology Information (NCBI)[Internet]. Bethesda (MD): National Library of Medicine (US), National Center for Biotechnology Information; [1988] – [cited 2024 May 18]. Available from: https://www.ncbi.nlm.nih.gov/pmc/articles/PMC6097542/

I was surprised once again. "They" tell us to take our vitamin C to not get sick. Yet here we are. Taking a form of mold which is linked to pneumonia and all kinds of other health issues. And then the B12 in your energy drinks and probably in the shots they give you as well. Remember from what we talked about earlier? Here's that receipt for you.

Vitamin B12 producing fermentations of sewage sludge origin with a mixed bacterium population. I. Role of individual bacterium species in vitamin B 12 production

National Center for Biotechnology Information (NCBI)[Internet]. Bethesda (MD): National Library of Medicine (US), National Center for Biotechnology Information; [1988] – [cited 2024 May 18]. Available from: https://pubmed.ncbi.nlm.nih.gov/5513795/#

The way I have begun to view foods, is that if it wasn't put here naturally, I don't want it. I have witnessed the power of the first step. The first day to say "no more." We can make this world better for ourselves by making our lives better.

If you ask a question one way, you get one answer. If you ask that same question in a different way, then you might get an entirely different answer. You might find that the people in charge debate themselves with their own findings and leave us to figure out what's right or wrong. For example, we are told food dyes are safe to consume. Then we find out they have all of these toxic effects on our bodies. We are told our laundry detergent is safe to use and then find it may leave chemicals on our skin that absorb into our bloodstream, and those chemicals, when ingested, cause neurological disorders and cancer, to name a few. Here are a few common contradictions I have found.

The FDA says it's safe.

Yes, color additives are safe when they are used in accordance with FDA regulations.

Nutrition, C. F. F. S. A. A. (2023, December 14). Color Additives Questions and Answers for Consumers. U.S. Food And Drug Administration. https://www.fda.gov/food/color-additives-information-consumers/color-additives-questions-and-answers-consumers#

Fun fact: Most of the food colors used in our foods and drinks are a by-product of the aluminum industry. And aluminum has had some pretty serious implications in our health decline as dementia and cancer studies are revealing.

Rd, B. B. M. (2023, July 17). Food Dyes: Harmless or Harmful? Healthline. https://www.healthline.com/nutrition/food-dyes#

In addition to considerations of organ damage, cancer, birth defects, and allergic reactions, mixtures of dyes (and Yellow 5 tested alone) cause hyperactivity and other behavioral problems in some children. Center for Science in the Public Interest. (2010, June). Food Dyes A Rainbow Of Risks. Retrieved May 18, 2024, from https://www.cspinet.org/sites/default/files/attachment/food-dyes-rainbow-of-risks.pdf

That is strange. I thought they said only red 3. If they lied about one...

This review I came across, finds that all of the nine currently US-approved dyes raise health concerns of varying degrees.

National Center for Biotechnology Information (NCBI)[Internet]. Bethesda (MD): National Library of Medicine (US), National Center for Biotechnology Information; [1988] – [cited 2024 May 18]. Available from: https://pubmed.ncbi.nlm.nih.gov/23026007/

WHAT THEY SAY: Sugar is not a carcinogenic (cancer-causing) substance. However, over-consumption of sugar, particularly added sugars in processed beverages and foods, can contribute to obesity which is an important risk factor for cancer. There is no evidence that consuming sugar makes cancer cells grow faster or cause cancer. Does sugar cause cancer? (n.d.). Cancer Council. https://www.cancer.org.au/iheard/does-sugar-cause-cancer

That Juice though: 5 Reasons Cancer Cells and Sugar Are Best Friends

D. (2021, April 16). *5 Reasons Cancer Cells and Sugar Are Best Friends*. Beat Cancer. https://beatcancer.org/blog/5-reasons-cancer-and-sugar-are-best-friends/

More Juice?

"My doctor cares" How western medicine lost its soul.

"Descartes dealt with this difficulty by splitting apart the body and the soul of man: he viewed the former as strictly mechanical and responsive to the directives of a separate spiritual soul by way of the pineal gland, a tiny structure inside the brain. His "ghost in the machine" metaphor still pervades the popular imagination to this day."

National Center for Biotechnology Information (NCBI)[Internet]. Bethesda (MD): National Library of Medicine (US), National Center for Biotechnology Information; [1988] – [cited 2024 May 18]. Available from: https://www.ncbi.nlm.nih.gov/pmc/articles/PMC5102204/#

"The government has agencies in place to protect us."

The Juice:" The United States government did something that was wrong -- deeply, profoundly, morally wrong. It was an outrage to our commitment to integrity and equality for all our citizens"

Apology For Study Done in Tuskegee. (n.d.).
https://clintonwhitehouse4.archives.gov/textonly/New/Remarks/Fri/19970516-898.html

This is from the White House apology speech on the Tuskegee experiment, when they gave 399 black men syphilis to examine the long-term effects without treatment. AND THEY DIDN'T TELL THEM THEY GAVE THEM SYPHILIS! JUST TO SEE WHAT HAPPENS!

Read! Question the motives. We are their experiment, it seems. Which takes us back toward the beginning of the book when I noted the Flexner report.

Flexner became adamant in his strive and polemics against all training facilities that offered education and postgraduate work in the above-mentioned fields and advocated for the closing of nearly eighty percent of all the contemporary programs in homeopathy, naturopathy, eclectic therapy, physical therapy, osteopathy, and chiropractic.

Unfortunately, Flexner may be rotating all too rapidly. [...] medical schools are teaching and promoting what is often called CAM, despite the lack of logic or evidence supporting many CAM practices.

Meanwhile, the same schools seem to give only lip service to the application of logic and evidence to healthcare, as exemplified by the formal processes of EBM. [49].

National Center for Biotechnology Information (NCBI)[Internet]. Bethesda (MD): National Library of Medicine (US), National Center for Biotechnology Information; [1988] – [cited 2024 May 18]. Available from: https://www.ncbi.nlm.nih.gov/pmc/articles/PMC3543812/#

By systematically limiting the extent of practice, notions of inferior black intellectual ability grew as blacks faced medical conditions, they were unable to treat.4 Flexner's attitude of helping blacks prepare themselves adequately for a restricted form of practice reinforced a concept of limited black ability.

National Center for Biotechnology Information (NCBI)[Internet]. Bethesda (MD): National Library of Medicine (US), National Center for Biotechnology Information; [1988] – [cited 2024 May 18]. Available from: https://www.ncbi.nlm.nih.gov/pmc/articles/PMC2571842/pdf/jnma00292-0091.pdf

How about this weather? It's like you can't look up in the sky without it being painted with the intricate cobwebs of death. Whose death may we be speaking of? Well, you of course. According to the:

OPERATIONAL PLAN FOR WEATHER MODIFICATION PROJECT WESTERN KANSAS WEATHER MODIFICATION 2014

All cloud base aircraft will be equipped with a Carley-type **silver iodide-acetone** burning generator mounted on each wing tip. The cloud base aircraft will operate from April 16th through September 15th, 2014. Each generator will dispense a three percent (by weight) silver iodide solution at a rate of (2.0 gallons per hour). All of the cloud base aircraft will also carry a special holding rack attached to the trailing edge of both wings, each of which is capable of carrying 12 pyrotechnic devices (flares) of the end-burning, burn-in-place variety.

These flares are designed to produce hygroscopic ice-forming nuclei, which promote the condensation-freezing-coalescence process within clouds.

Based on studies of weather modification programs in states such as California, Colorado, Arizona, Texas, Florida and both South and North Dakota.

Submitted to:(1) Chairman, WKGMD#1 (2) Director, KWO (3) Director, Colorado Water Board (4) Oklahoma Water Resources Board

WESTERN KANSAS GROUNDWATER MANAGEMENT DISTRICT NO. 1. (2014). OPERATIONAL PLAN FOR WEATHER MODIFICATION PROJECT WESTERN KANSAS WEATHER MODIFICATION 2014. Retrieved May 30, 2024, from https://library.oarcloud.noaa.gov/noaa_documents.lib/OAR/OWAQ/Weather_Modification_Project/Operational%20Plan%20For%20Weather%20Modification%20Project%20-%20Western%20Kansas%20Weather%20Modification%202014.pdf

Don't worry. I read it. The report says we're okay. There's no signs of risk to health or land or blah, blah, blah. The usual lies we're being told as we're being poisoned. You know I kept going. From various sources across the web, the side effects of over exposure to silver iodide-acetone include:

- **Nausea and vomiting**
- **Lack of coordination**
- **Coma**
- **Difficulty breathing**
- **Drowsiness**
- **Headache**
- **Loss of consciousness**
- **Confusion**
- **Irritation/Rash**
- **Person may have a fruity odor**
- **Slowed breathing rate**

- **Cough**
- **Dizziness**
- **Sore throat**

Unfortunately, that did not suffice my appetite. I know we are not being told the truth. I had to do some digging. And of course I found it in the national Library of medicine. Ag is the element symbol for silver. So, you know.

4.4. The Ag^+ from the APE will cause risk to the environment and drink water source

Though the Ag^+ concentration in the water increase by 42.86 %, this concentration was still far below the Ag^+ content threshold of the drinking water in China. However, three risks to the environment and ecosystem which the Ag^+ from the APE may bring should not be neglected. First, the residual Ag^+ from the APE in the air could become a new aerosol pollutant, that could drift away to other areas by floating in the air and this may bring damage to the ecosystem of other areas where the APE was not conducted. Second, soil serves as a bank of Ag^+ originating from APE, as extensive Ag^+ accumulate in the soil following continuous APE activities. These Ag^+ ions may be absorbed by plants and bring harm to their growth, Subsequently, animals would also be affected if they ate the polluted plants since Ag^+ can accumulate in the brain [27]. Through precipitation and soil erosion, the Ag^+ may be transferred to other places that may negatively influence to the ecosystems, specifically, agricultural ecosystem. Additionally, fungi and other microorganisms may potentially be damaged by the external Ag^+ [[65], [66], [67]], Ag^+ may lead to the destruction of the respiratory chain of cells [68], bind to sulfhydryl or other proteins, and inhibit the enzyme activity of bacteria involved in the phosphorus, sulfur, and nitrogen cycles [[69], [70], [71], [72], [73]], This can inactivate microorganisms [74]. At the same time, both nitrifying microorganisms and ammonia oxidation rates in soil may be negatively affected [75]. On the other hand, Ag^+ penetrates the cell membrane into the cell interior and can inhibit cell division and destroy DNA replication [[76], [77], [78], [79], [80], [81]]. Soil microorganisms are an important component of farmland ecosystems and an important index for maintaining soil fertility and crop production [82]. Therefore, silver ions will inevitably affect soil productivity on the premise that they affect soil microorganisms. The decline of soil productivity also leads to the destruction of soil ecosystems. The Ag^+ in the soil may combine with other ions, such as cupric ions, and then produce toxic pollutants. Meanwhile, Ag^+ is also an important catalyst for causing other types of pollution [83]. Third, our study indicates that the water body can adjust the concentration of Ag^+ over the long term to ensure that the content does not become very high; however these Ag^+ may be deposited in the bottom soil of the water body. This may generate a long-term Ag^+ release source and cause a substantial g risk to the drinking water source.

Data availability statement

The data associated with the study has not been deposited into any publicly available repository. It will be made available **on** request.

I wonder why they haven't made this publicly available? I bet the medical field may know. Well, don't worry. I'll help. Sorry Dick. I MEAN JOHN.

I hope that reading this will encourage you to ask more questions and get more involved in your health. Simply by being more aware of the poisons that are in our foods and killing us every day. Since I began this journey, I have stopped and helped as much as possible. But if everyone could understand that as soon as you take your first step, your life changes.

From my experience, the first day I took sea moss, the colors of our world became more vibrant. The grass was truly greener in my vision. The sky is more of a vibrant blue. I cannot explain how good it feels to come back alive again. After working as a mechanic for 20 years, my hair was thinning and graying. My body hurt often, and I didn't realize how bad I was doing until I started taking all of this to support my wife. It turns out, I needed to get myself healthy as well. Since then, my hair has thickened up a bit and is actually losing the gray instead. My wife's constantly getting compliments on her hair, skin and nails. They all started responding like crazy. Her hair grows faster and her nails naturally feel like acrylics because they are that strong and healthy. Please, if you are buying foods that have chemicals in them you can't pronounce, stop buying them. This is nonsense. Our "food" is not food anymore. It's some man-made chemicals mixed together that they have sold to us as food. Allow me to tie this together with what should be my master thesis: Although the government and many horrible people have coerced us into doing this to ourselves, i.e., giving ourselves cancer, tumors, Alzheimer's, obesity, etc., for profit, they cannot get away with it forever. People from Abraham Flexner and Herman Gates Weiskotten, to our own modern-day masterminds.

The United States Corporation's Food and Drug Administration seems to be attacking us through our food sources with misinformation and a very seemingly ill intent for the living souls on this plane. It seems we are obviously abhorred.

Please allow me to leave you with these two final points:

First: It is important to consider the fact that Hippocrates, who is considered to be the father of clinical medicine, said, "Let food be thy medicine, and medicine be thy food.".

National Center for Biotechnology Information (NCBI)[Internet]. Bethesda (MD): National Library of Medicine (US), National Center for Biotechnology Information; [1988] – [cited 2024 May 18]. Available from: https://pubmed.ncbi.nlm.nih.gov/19567383/

With the facts in hand, I leave you with second and final point.

If you have asked yourself why doesn't the government stop this? Do they know? Has it been presented in their current required format in a way they can understand? Yes, it has.

The crème de la crème. I have found in my research and studies, documentation from the National Library of Medicine and it states that the U.S. government is having to publicly acknowledge all of the facts that you've learned while reading this book. And simultaneously, still they are allowing money and lobbying to undermine and disregard us as living men and women. A report by the WORLD HEALTH ORGANIZATION backing up the fact that our foods can prevent chronic disease:

The question of fortifying foods inevitably becomes highly political, and the politics of nutrition are just as complex as the science. Owen Dyer tells how the United States government—lobbied by food manufacturers—is trying to undermine a report by the World Health Organization on Diet, Nutrition, and the Prevention of Chronic Disease (p 185).

National Center for Biotechnology Information (NCBI)[Internet]. Bethesda (MD): National Library of Medicine (US), National Center for Biotechnology Information; [1988] – [cited 2024 May 18]. Available from: https://www.ncbi.nlm.nih.gov/pmc/articles/PMC318470/

They know. They simply and obviously do not care. Ballentine's Law Dictionary defines treason as a *breach of allegiance by one who owes allegiance, perpetual or temporary.*

I thought they worked for us? Have they violated the 1925 Geneva Protocol against the poisoning of humans? Let there be no doubt in your mind that you are being poisoned. It's only by whom? That is the Question. Is it you? Or them? They lie to us and then sell it. We buy it. Know that:

The International committee of the Red Cross (ICRC) considers any use of biological agents to cause illness, death, or fear to be utterly repugnant and abhorrent. Such acts deserve universal condemnation, especially as they are banned by the 1925 Geneva Protocol, 1972 Biological Weapons Convention.

Rules prohibiting poisoning and deliberate spread of disease. (n.d.). ICRC.
https://www.icrc.org/en/doc/resources/documents/misc/5vdjfc.htm#

We want to know how they claim this right over us to commit these atrocities. The answers are out there. Question everything. If you don't like your answer. Reformulate the question. Computers can only lie to you or should I say "mis-guide" you so much and so far. Questions like: Why do you have a social security number anyway? Well, another way to ask or search that information, one would need to research: THE STORY OF THE BUCK ACT by Richard McDonald. This was an interesting find indeed. Oops.

E. (n.d.). Wheeling Steel Corp v. Fox – Freedom Documents. Freedom Documents.
https://keystoliberty2.wordpress.com/tag/wheeling-steel-corp-v-fox/

Thank you for coming along on this journey. I hope you have gained a small world of knowledge. In the end I believe we were both lucky and strategic. I believe we still need doctors and their equipment. I just think we need to keep our minds extremely aware of our new found comprehension of the medical field and what they truly are doing to us. Always know your truth. Whatever that may be. This once again is not medical advice. This is merely a compilation of information that I came across in the middle of the night, trying to find the way to save my wife. I suggest anyone reading this to do their own research. Draw your own conclusions. If you would like to show support, it is always appreciated and can be shown on cashapp at $killinghercancer the QR is linked below. Reach out if you feel necessary, Contact@killinghercancer.com It is now 3:42 a.m. and I am going to bed. As with all of my research, this too was written and edited in the middle of the night. I will leave you with the only advice I have to give. If you have found any grammatical errors, keep them to yourself. If you have the options, please shop at a local butcher. Find a local nursery, or shop at a farmers' market. It all started with this first step you have already just taken, upon the reading of this book. Further your education any way that you can. Eat better foods. Drink better water. Live better. Love yourself.

Live well my friends,

Guero

S. Heinson

Killing Her Cancer
Scan to pay $killinghercancer

contact@killinghercancer.com

hardpressedlife.com

P.S. 9 months after her tumor was reduced to 0mm and no detectable traces were remaining, we discovered that she had a couple of small benign tumors in her breast. Which were successfully removed in a partial mastectomy. I must note that breast cancer is often misdiagnosed in its early stages. Always get a second opinion. Regardless, they were benign. Incapable of growing further due to her internal environment that was successfully maintained in an alkaline state. Verified by her ph. tests. Although I don't have more information as far as growth patterns or time as they were removed upon discovery. No chances were going to be taken. We've already gone down that road!

:S:

www.ingramcontent.com/pod-product-compliance
Lightning Source LLC
Chambersburg PA
CBHW070929270326
41927CB00011B/2788